HEALING WITH THE
MIND'S EYE

Other Books by Michael Samuels

With Mary Rockwood Lane

Spirit Body Healing: Using Your Mind's Eye to Unlock the Medicine Within

Shaman Wisdom, Shaman Healing: Deepen Your Ability to Heal with Visionary and Spiritual Tools and Practices

Creative Healing: How to Heal Yourself by Tapping Your Inner Creativity

The Path of the Feather: A Handbook and Kit for Making Medicine Wheels and Calling in the Spirit Animals

With Nancy Samuels

Seeing with the Mind's Eye

The Well Baby Book

The Well Child Book

The Well Child Coloring Book

The Well Pregnancy Book

The Well Adult

Take Charge of Your Hypertension

Take Charge of Your Arthritis

Take Charge of Your Heart Disease

With Hal Z. Bennett

The Well Body Book

Spirit Guides: Access to Inner Worlds

Be Well

Well Body, Well Earth

HEALING WITH THE MIND'S EYE

HOW TO USE GUIDED IMAGERY AND VISIONS TO HEAL BODY, MIND, AND SPIRIT

Revised and Updated Edition

Michael Samuels, M.D.

WILEY

John Wiley & Sons, Inc.

Published by John Wiley & Sons, Inc., Hoboken, New Jersey
Published simultaneously in Canada

Design and production by Navta Associates, Inc.

For general information about our other products and services, please contact our Customer Care Department within the United States at (800) 762-2974, outside the United States at (317) 572-3993 or fax (317) 572-4002.

Wiley also publishes its books in a variety of electronic formats. Some content that appears in print may not be available in electronic books. For more information about Wiley products, visit our web site at www.wiley.com.

Library of Congress Cataloging-in-Publication Data:

Samuels, Michael, M.D.
  Healing with the mind's eye : how to use guided imagery and visions to heal body, mind, and spirit, revised and updated edition / Michael Samuels.
     p. cm.
  Previously published: New York : Summit Books, c1990.
  Includes bibliographical references and index.
  ISBN 0-471-45908-9 (pbk.)
     1. Imagery (Psychology)—Therapeutic use. 2. Imagination—Therapeutic use. 3. Maturation (Psychology) 4. Self-actualization (Psychology) I. Title.

RC489.F35S26   2003
616.89'14—dc21   2003053800

Printed in the United States of America

ISBN 978-1-63026-099-6 (hc)

To Nancy and her everlasting love

CONTENTS

PREFACE

It is with great pleasure that I give you this new edition of *Healing with the Mind's Eye*. The book is beloved to me and many patients; it has often been referenced as a basic guided imagery sourcebook. Its deep and powerful guided imagery exercises are transformative and healing. We have had numerous requests for a new edition and are delighted that John Wiley & Sons and Tom Miller, my editor, have made it happen.

The material in *Healing with the Mind's Eye* is as revolutionary today as it was when it was written ten years ago; there is little in the book that I have changed. *Healing with the Mind's Eye* was ahead of its time when it was published: guided imagery and spiritual techniques are now in the forefront of medicine. Medicine has changed, and guided imagery's role in health care has changed. Guided imagery has gone from a new unproven technique to a powerful research-proven tool that is now in use in most hospitals. The guided imagery exercises in *Healing with the Mind's Eye* are among the most detailed and advanced guided imagery exercises available.

Medicine is catching up with *Healing with the Mind's Eye* in its approach to healing the whole person—body, mind, and spirit. Medicine today strives to look at the patient as a whole. The mission statement for many leading medical centers is stated clearly, you even hear it on the radio in publicity and promotion releases. "Our goal is to treat the whole person—body, mind, and spirit." There are now seventy-five departments of spirituality and health care in major medical centers, including several with multimillion-dollar grants and budgets from the National Institutes of Health (NIH). The most forward-thinking health theorists teach us that we are more than our bodies, and that healing the spirit or the soul increases healing by 100 percent. Some health care theorists even call soul or spirit healing the 100 percent factor.

When asking about what a physician has done to heal a patient, they ask, "Did you use the 100 percent factor; did you heal spirit?"

Patients are different now, too. They are more creative, they are interested in the earth, personal growth, consciousness, meditation, and spirituality. They want to be healed as well as cured. They want to learn and be changed by an illness experience, they want to grow and expand their consciousness. They want their suffering to inform their existence. Thinking of illness as a purely negative experience has been replaced by thinking of it as an opportunity for change and transformation. *Healing with the Mind's Eye* explains how to make illness transformative in a person's life. It gives people tools to expand their consciousness and grow in each guided imagery exercise. If you come to this book with an illness, you will learn how to take your illness and use it to create deep change. After healing, you can make your life more beautiful than you have ever dreamed.

New research in guided imagery has validated the initial expectations about how imagery effects physiology and health. Guided imagery is now known as the magic bullet in body, mind, and spirit medicine. It is used in almost every body-mind intervention. For the body, the latest research indicates that guided imagery decreases headache pain in tension headache patients, decreases anxiety and pain in surgical patients, shortens hospital stay and reduces medication use in post-surgical heart surgery and colon surgery patients. This last research alone demonstrates that guided imagery would save an average hospital millions of dollars a year and mandates that every hospital put a guided imagery program into surgical units.

Guided imagery has also been shown to reduce the side effects of chemotherapy and radiation in cancer patients, reduce blood glucose levels in diabetics, reduce allergy symptoms, and enhance sleep. This research gives each of us the impetus to use guided imagery for healing. The guided imagery exercises in this book are as powerful as most medications used for healing and pain relief.

For the mind, guided imagery has been shown in numerous studies to enhance self-confidence and self-esteem and to enhance a person's total quality of life. Guided imagery has been shown in randomized studies to be a catalyst for spiritual experiences and growth. If there was a medication that could do even a part of this body, mind, and spirit healing, it would be hailed as the largest medical breakthrough of the century. Indeed, guided imagery is that breakthrough.

Welcome to this new edition of *Healing with the Mind's Eye.* New readers are welcomed and are invited on this exciting journey of healing. Use the 100 percent factor to optimize your healing. Heal your body, mind, and spirit with the wonderful research-proven techniques in this book.

ACKNOWLEDGMENTS

I feel a deep sense of gratitude to patients and workshop participants I have worked with over my many years of practice. From them, I have learned the beauty and dignity of healing.

I also wish to thank a number of colleagues who have profoundly affected my thought and practice. For the first edition I want to thank Jeanne Achterberg and Frank Lawlis, who have been mentors to me and many others. Our workshops together have been moving and transformative. I want to thank Michael Lerner and all the staff at Commonweal for showing me how love and healing can coexist with technical medical treatment. Special thanks to all the people who have participated in the Symington Foundation Conferences on New Directions in Cancer Care. I value each of them for their knowledge and their openness. I also wish to thank my dear friends Phyllis and Marshall Klaus, from whom I've benefited greatly by exchanging ideas about healing.

Books do not appear magically by themselves. For this book's existence I owe special appreciation to my agent, Elaine Markson, and her associate, Geri Toma, who have understood this project from the beginning; to my original editor, Dominick Anfuso, for his thoughtful review of the manuscript; and to my original publisher, Jim Silberman, for his support over close to twenty years. I would like to thank Tom Miller, my editor at Wiley, for his insight in bringing this book back to us all.

Finally I would like to thank my family: my sons, Rudy and Lewis, for their love and support; my sister, Linda, who read this manuscript and gave valuable suggestions about using the exercises; my nephew, Wen, who kept my computers working; my parents, for their continued love. For this second edition I want to thank the Spirituality and Healthcare Group at the University of Florida; and Mary Rockwood Lane, for sharing her knowledge of creativity, spirituality, and healing with me for the last ten years.

PART ONE

JOY AND DELIGHT— AH-H

INTRODUCTION

Happiness, Health, and the Healing Spirit

You can enhance your own healing: You can act to help make yourself well. *Healing with the Mind's Eye* is a book about healing, change, and transformation, a book that can help you find intense power in moments of weakness and courage in moments of fear. Deep within yourself right now, you have the power to heal yourself and to grow. This book will help make that inner strength available to you by giving you knowledge and techniques through which you can go inward and change the way you look at the world. That new perception will alter the physiology of your immune system and will change your attitude. Images and visions are not difficult to understand or use; they are the stuff of daydreams, creativity, and prayer. People use imagery techniques every day, but they rarely take advantage of them intentionally for growth or healing. Using imagery to travel inward to a new world of beauty and excitement is an extraordinary experience.

I am a physician who has specialized in helping people use guided imagery for healing and personal growth. For more than thirty years I have worked with guided imagery, and I have found it to be a powerful tool for healing. I became interested in guided imagery through the study of yoga during college, and hypnosis during my residency. I first used guided imagery in medicine when I cofounded Headlands Clinic, a holistic medical practice, in 1969. In 1975 I coauthored *Seeing with the Mind's Eye,* the first major book on guided imagery and healing, with my wife, Nancy. Since that time, the field of guided imagery has grown and flourished, and guided imagery has become an established complementary therapy in medicine. It is used in many conditions, including cancer, heart disease, AIDS, and arthritis. Guided imagery is now used in coordination with other therapies, including surgery, radiation, and drugs. It is often part of a therapeutic plan that includes nutrition, exercise, herbs, and so on. People develop a group of healing actions that appeal to them and that they believe in. Guided imagery is particularly easy to use and effective. The guided imagery experiences in this book are designed to enhance healing. Clinical experience has shown that everyone can benefit from guided imagery. I have found that people can help themselves heal and grow, and can improve their lives immeasurably. We are all the same; we all share the same hopes and fears. Guided imagery can help turn fear into hope.

For the last several years I have taught guided imagery in many different types of workshops. Some workshops were for patients with life-threatening illnesses, some were for people with life problems, and some were training workshops for physicians, nurses, and other health care providers. I started teaching workshops because many people wanted to learn more about guided imagery, especially people who had cancer. They became interested in guided imagery through their doctor's recommendations, through word of mouth, and through other books. I like the idea of working with groups because most participants develop a sense of increased connectedness, support, and power. In the workshops I found that basic information about imagery, combined with imagery exercises, was most effective. I developed a series of exercises that I found to be exciting and powerful. These exercises involved increased use of visions and a feeling of sacred connectedness to a force greater than one's own personality. For me, these new exercises energized the guided imagery process and added a life that had been missing. People who came to the workshops often felt a sense of increased power, a lessening of symptoms, and a sense of renewal and growth. Some were healed of life-threatening illnesses.

Guided imagery can help you in several ways. First, relaxation techniques and guided imagery have been shown in research studies to affect the body's physiology. They can enhance the immune system, which defends the body against viruses and bacteria and even cancer cells. Guided imagery can lower blood pressure and heart rate, which is useful in treating and preventing heart disease. Guided imagery can decrease pain and alleviate the side effects of many drugs, including chemotherapy. Second, guided imagery profoundly affects attitude. It can increase feelings of confidence, control, and power, and decrease hopelessness, depression, and fear. These changes in attitude have been shown to enhance healing as well. There is also some evidence that support can extend life for cancer patients. Finally, guided imagery is an age-old tool for personal and spiritual growth. Guided imagery can help people solve life problems and make important choices. Guided imagery helps us realize that we are connected to the world around us and are part of the earth's power. This sense of interconnection gives us the ability to create, to balance, and to make a better world. It makes us feel good in the moment and helps us to love life and the world around us.

Healing with the Mind's Eye has three goals: happiness, health, and the healing spirit. In *happiness*, we will help you feel hope and joy in the moment; in *health*, we will help you prevent illness, relieve discomfort, and enhance healing; and in *spirit*, we will help you feel at peace with the world, help you communicate with your inner self to feel the force that underlies all nature and healing.

If you have an illness, the main goal of the book is to enhance your healing. I will endeavor to help you create a positive attitude filled with enthusiasm and faith. I have used guided imagery with people who have had many types of illness, including cancer, AIDS, multiple sclerosis, arthritis, and heart disease, and I have seen these people's lives improve greatly. People I have worked with have healed from life-threatening illness. If you have a friend or a loved one who has an illness, this book can give you the strength and special skills to help that person change. It can give you energy to share with him or her.

If you seek personal growth, I will try to help you learn about yourself and your path in order to achieve clarity and reassurance. Our goal will be to build guided imagery skills that will help you make decisions and choices that will connect you to the flow of life. I have used these exercises with many people who are trying to solve problems and make important decisions, and I know they are transformative.

Healing with the Mind's Eye is divided into two parts. The first part, "Joy and Delight," introduces you to the basic tool, the guided imagery process, and to the effect that spirit has on mind and that mind has on body. The second part of the book, "Healing in the Sacred Space," gives you practice in using this technique to heal body, mind, and spirit. The feeling of the first part of the book is "ah-h," the sound of enjoyment and awakening. This part of the book is designed to be a wonderful experience. The feeling of the second part of the book is "peace"; it is the sound of silence or awe before a greater power than ourselves. The feeling of this part of the book is the feeling of deep healing.

In Part One we allow the guided imagery process to change us. In Chapter 1 I'll talk about how the spirit heals. The first exercise will start us on the healing path and will introduce us to the feeling of guided imagery. In Chapter 2 I will talk about the inner world and how it feels. The exercises in Chapter 2 are the basic exercises needed to start working with guided imagery. In Chapter 3, "The Journey," I'll talk about the tremendous power that positive attitudes can have on health. The exercises for Chapter 3 will take us deeper into guided imagery and help us clarify our own personal myth. In Chapter 4, the last chapter of Part One, I'll talk about inner guides. In the exercises in Chapter 4 we'll practice meeting and talking with our own guides.

In Part Two of the book we will actively work with images and visions as healing tools. In Chapter 5 I will define sacred space and talk about light as a healing image. The exercise for this chapter involves feeling the sacred space and seeing white light. In Chapter 6, "The Vision," I will discuss creating healing visions with guides and creating a mythological adventure. The exercises for this chapter will show how to use guides and visions for healing. In Chapter 7, "The Image," I will deal with using guided imagery for healing specific illnesses or problems. The exercises will involve creating and practicing healing imagery and feeling healing energy. The final chapter, Chapter 8, will deal with the relationship between spiritual transformation and healing. The exercises in Chapter 8 will consist of an ascendant vision. This chapter will complete our journey and help us bring our inner tools out to the world.

Each chapter is divided into three parts. The first part contains the knowledge that makes choices possible. The more knowledge we have about how body, mind, and spirit work, the clearer we are about what is important in our lives and the less likely we are to be misled. To effect change through knowledge takes study and reflection. Often, information is assimilated slowly and must be digested, thought over, criticized, and questioned. We absorb those ideas that intuitively make sense to us, that ring a bell or turn on a light in our minds. The new ideas that we incorporate alter the way we look at the world and help us change.

The second part of each chapter is a discussion that introduces the exercises and reassures you about what it is like to do them. It addresses questions that are often asked in workshops and discusses in detail the feelings that characterize the experience. The third part of each chapter consists of exercises that are meant to be experienced. Simply experiencing the exercises will bring about change by itself. Unlike the slow change produced by knowledge, the change brought about by the exercises is spontaneous and automatic. The transformation occurs at a deep level in our unconscious, below the level of conscious thought and evaluation. We do not need to do anything to effect this change other than to deeply experience the exercise. Whereas change through knowledge takes reflection, change through experience takes practice, doing the exercise slowly, and giving yourself plenty of time. For most people this involves about ten hours of total exercise time and is best spread over a week or several weeks. Experiencing the exercises more and more deeply produces profound transformation. When images or symbols are released from the unconscious, new pathways are opened in the mind, allowing our body to heal.

Healing with the Mind's Eye is an unusual book because it is intended to be both a personal experience and a two-way communication. While I'm speaking to you, I hope you will take time to stop and think over the material, to ask yourself questions, and to receive answers from your inner self. In the quiet of your mind, speak back. I also hope that the book will be more than something to read; I hope it will become something to experience and feel. If you come to this book with openness and the intent to change, it will happen, and it will come about by itself. You need only to listen and try the exercises. I've found these exercises to be magical; they can help move you into the unknown and let your spirit soar. If you spend time on the exercises, you will be different at the end of this book.

People that I have worked with have healed illness, increased hope, moved from depression to joy, relieved pain, learned about themselves, made important decisions, and rediscovered a desire to live. Guided imagery can do these things for you. A woman with metastatic breast cancer came to a workshop upset and on edge. She felt that everything was out of control and that nothing positive existed in her life. After learning imagery and beginning her exercises, she changed. She regained her sense of humor, and her pain lessened dramatically. She began to smile and looked beautiful. The group loved her, and she helped everyone. She was full of joy and love. Her life changed. Let us awaken and start our journey. Let us begin to travel inward. Let us begin to help ourselves heal.

1

THE AWAKENING

I believe that images and visions have enormous power and that images freed from our inner center can change us profoundly. I believe that when an image emerges, we glimpse the energy of the universe, and our souls are fed. In my own life and in my work with patients and people in workshops, I have seen the healing spirit emerge from deep inside people, and I have watched them as they grew and flourished.

Each of us can draw on our profound abilities to enhance our own healing. In many instances we can even heal serious or chronic illnesses, including those that may not usually be curable. Much of our ability to heal results from empowerment and control. By changing our attitudes and worldview we can take control of our lives and free our body's healing abilities to work at their best. This is a book about letting images connect us with something greater and realign mind, body, and spirit. When body, mind, and spirit act as one, optimum healing can occur.

When I teach in workshops or work with people who have an illness, my goal is to create a space of healing, which I believe is sacred space. People who come to me wish to solve the problems in their lives, or they have an illness that they are struggling to deal with. Many of the illnesses are life-threatening, and the people are frightened and depressed. I hope when you finish this book you will begin to heal: you will look and feel younger and stronger; you will let worry leave your face and bring energy back into your step; you will solve problems, get answers, relieve symptoms; and you will feel better. I hope you will heal and live a long, full rich life. I have written this book to resemble a series of workshop sessions or one-to-one patient visits in which I will speak to each of you personally. But since I am not there physically, my voice and presence can be with you. The energy of healing will come to you through my words and intent.

The ultimate goal of this book is to help us heal ourselves and grow by rediscovering a part of our consciousness that in many of us lies dormant. Human consciousness is as multifaceted as a precious gem. It contains aspects that participate in outer reality, make decisions, and meet everyday needs. It also contains parts that reach for creative ideas, seek deep connections with other people, and strive to understand spiritual realities. I believe that the part of our consciousness that is creative and knows spiritual union helps to heal our mind, body, and spirit. It has been called the Self, the soul, the spirit, or the inner center. All of us have this spiritual core within us. However, many of us have not been taught to look upon illness and healing from this point of view. When we become ill and go to a doctor, most often the doctor approaches the problem in a mechanistic way, and so do we. We see our body—a physical entity—responding to drugs or surgery—also physical entities. I believe that the situation is far more complex. The mind and spirit play an important part in protecting and healing the body. It is now known that the mind actually sends out messages and substances that control the remarkable ability of the immune system to surround and destroy viruses and cancer cells. This is an important part of our body's subtle and complex means of producing healing.

If you have an illness, I see this book as an important part of your medical treatment. It will supplement whatever drugs, radiation, and surgical treatments you are receiving and strengthen these treatments by changing your attitudes, by giving you the skills, imagery, and visions to free your body's own healing mechanisms. Although age-old, guided imagery is new to modern medicine. Guided imagery simply involves picturing scenes in your mind's eye. The mental images affect the nervous system, the immune system, and the physiology of the whole body, and ultimately enhance healing. Specific guided imagery techniques are now widely used in many fields of medicine and are an accepted therapy for many serious conditions, including cancer and AIDS. Guided imagery is used to prepare patients for surgery and to prepare them for procedures. If you do not have an illness, you will find the experience of this book to be equally powerful. We all face problems in our lives; this is the human condition. Guided imagery skills can apply to any type of life change or problem; they are not limited to illness. In this book, the word "healing" is synonymous with growth and transformation.

At a certain level, healing comes from our hearts. All of us can enhance our own healing—we can make ourselves feel better, and we can increase our control over symptoms and illnesses. That is not to say that we can live forever or completely cure all illnesses. But we know that people can improve their lives immeasurably by actively participating in their healing. And many people who have used imagery have cured themselves of illnesses that were life-threatening or said to be incurable. All of us working in the field of imagery have different beliefs and experiences in relation to guided imagery's ability to extend life. Although everyone agrees that people can improve their lives immeasurably with guided imagery, the question of longevity is still unproven. Many physicians and psychologists who work with guided imagery and life-threatening illnesses estimate that imagery helps cure between 10 and 40 percent of people who would not be expected to live on the basis of medical therapy alone. But these figures are currently based on the personal experience of individual healers and have not been documented in controlled studies.

One research study has shown that a psychological approach can affect the survival of cancer patients. Dr. David Spiegel, from the Department of Psychiatry and Behavioral Sciences at Stanford, randomly assigned eighty-six women with metastatic breast cancer to one of two groups. Both groups received standard medical treatment, but the experimental group also had a year of weekly group support sessions, one part of which was learning self-hypnotic techniques. The group also discussed their illness, their treatment, and their personal concerns. Much of their discussion centered on facing death and dying. Over time, the group came to love and support each other outside of the therapy sessions, as well as within. On average, the women who went to the support sessions lived nearly twice as long after the study began as the women who did not participate in the support groups. They experienced half the pain, and had less mood disturbance. This study strongly suggests that psychological approaches affect longevity, but larger and more conclusive studies are needed. Whether or not guided imagery is conclusively proven to affect longevity (as I believe it will be), guided imagery improves the quality of life and reduces pain and the side effects of treatment, and thus is valuable in and of itself.

I believe that the spirit frees the mind to heal the body, that by journeying inward we can reach that place of healing. By experiencing states of consciousness similar to creative and religious experiences, we can align body, mind, and spirit and cause a transformation that heals our body. Thus I see healing as an inner journey, and its beginning as an awakening. In a workshop, transformation takes place during the imagery journeys that people undertake. The work is personal and takes place within their minds and spirits. Patients and workshop participants may find that they initially feel strange when they are doing the exercises for the first time. But almost everyone is enriched by the experience. Everyone can listen to stories and picture faraway places; we can all remember being on beaches or in the mountains, and can almost feel the sun or wind on our skin. Doing guided imagery exercises simply involves letting our imagination travel; it is like directed daydreaming. We all daydream about pleasurable experiences, even during work. In this book, we will use the power of the image to help us heal.

I like to begin any healing journey with a brief exercise that helps to alter our focus and to make us aware of our concerns in a broader perspective. I have found that starting with a daydream-like rest relaxes us, changes our state of mind, and is a good introduction to the work ahead. For this experience, you can either image as you read or read the exercise first, then lie down, close your eyes, and go over it in your mind. Simply let the experience happen. The exercise is a giving thanks, and a request like a prayer.

Take several deep breaths and let yourself relax. Imagine that you are in a clearing in the country at dusk on a warm, clear evening. You have journeyed here from a distance to join in a healing experience. You may be either a healer or a person with an illness, or both. Feel the ground beneath you, smell the air, and look at the stars above. Imagine you are seated on the ground in a circle of familiar people. In your mind, look around at the people in the circle and feel the goodness and love in each person. You may recognize friends, relatives, or healers that you know. Or you may feel connections to people in the circle for reasons that you are unaware of.

Now, give thanks for your life. Give thanks for the support of your loved ones and healers. Imagine that a feeling of love and healing energy fills the clearing. As you welcome the healing energy, let it flow through your body. Feel the force from which the energy comes. It may be from the earth, from the sky, or from a supreme power. Allow a specific request for help to come into your mind; it can be a request for healing, for knowledge, for help with a problem in your life. The important thing is to ask for something. Acknowledge the help you will receive with a sense of thankfulness or, if you wish, a brief prayer. The prayer may be one that you make up or one that you have learned in the past that has special meaning for you. Rest in the space that you have created. Enjoy the feelings of healing energy that you share with the group.

How did this exercise make you feel? Did you have unexpected thoughts or images? Did you simply feel somewhat different from usual? This brief exercise was a guided imagery experience. I realize that it may be new to you and may even have felt strange. Some people have a daydream when they read the exercise, others simply relax, and still others may feel frustrated by their lack of images. Don't worry about how you felt doing this first exercise. It was only a brief introduction to guided imagery. This book will teach you to picture and experience images deeply. Step by step, it will make this powerful skill useful to you for healing and personal growth.

In any group situation or workshop, it's valuable to begin by having the participants in the circle introduce themselves. This sharing is inspiring and helps people focus on their own reasons for being there, both known and unrealized. Although a book is very different from a workshop, a reader can experience some of the same effects that are produced by a group's energy. In this book, however, the group must be imaginary, which may make the task somewhat more difficult. It is often useful for readers to create an imaginary group that surrounds and supports them while they're using the book. To do this, mentally list those family members, friends, acquaintances, and healers that you want to be in your group. You can simply imagine such a group, or you might even wish to talk to those people about your healing work. In workshops, we refer to this as "calling in your ancestors." You allow images of people—real or imaginary—who have helped you in your life to come to mind. You may have glimpsed your group during the brief exercise, or you may have previously worked with a group in a workshop that you can use now.

I believe that all the people reading this book are remarkable because they are more open than many people, more likely to take active charge of their lives and health, and more likely to look for novel solutions to problems. Finally, whether they would say so or not, they are more likely to have an interest in inner or spiritual concerns. From the outset, all of these characteristics are healing ones. Among the people who read this book, many will already have progressed far on their healing journey. It's worthwhile to reflect on the progress that has already been made; personal introductions allow people to see where they have been. Since we will be in close contact for some time, it is valuable for you to have some idea of who I am. Look at this introduction as a personal meeting. Try to imagine that I am with you and talking to you. Here is my introduction:

I see myself as a person who's always been interested in healing and in images. From the youngest age, I was interested in doctors, doctors' offices, and the magic that I believed took place there. At the same time, as a child in my pediatrician's office, I felt that the healing that went on there resulted from an interaction between the doctor and the patient and had something to do with an energy that passed between them. I did not know what was happening, but I felt that the doctor's office was different from other places. It was more serious and real; there was an excitement about it that felt alive. As a child, I felt as if faith, belief, mystery, and the unknown had much to do with the healing situation. Even when I was young I felt that I would be a doctor, but I knew I would be different from the kind of doctors I had met. For one thing, the atmosphere of doctors' offices was not warm and supportive; it was scary, even though the doctor might not have been frightening. Mostly I found that doctors did not deal with the real concerns and problems I had. I had a feeling that the doctor was the figure in society who should deal with the problems that I intuited were the cause of my illness.

My other great interest as a child was photography. Making images on paper became my passion. The quiet space and energy around the making of each picture was exhilarating and took me to a different place in my mind. After school I would wander in the country and spend hours taking photographs of dry grass in the snow or reflections on water. Immediately before taking each picture, I would feel as if I were in a timeless space where all thought ceased. In my darkroom at night I would enter the same space when I saw the picture slowly emerge on the paper. I knew that my pictures were healing to me. In my photography I could somehow create an energy and feeling similar to the healing situation I yearned for in the doctor's office. Looking back on my photography, I now feel that the energy of creating art is the same as the energy of healing. Both bring you into your creative center, and both make you feel more alive.

In high school and college my interest in healing caused me to participate in research projects and to plan to go to medical school. I thought then that my path lay in research, and I spent my time investigating the ability of the lymphocyte, a special type of white blood cell, to produce antibodies. But research was not fulfilling enough for me; something personal and spiritual was missing. At that point immunology was not associated with the mind, and the research somehow seemed cold and empty. During medical school I married Nancy Harrison, whom I had met in college. In her I saw a loving, giving person, someone with whom I could share my life.

During my residency I had the good fortune to study with Dr. David Cheek, an obstetrician/gynecologist who used hypnotherapy as a major tool in his medical practice. Watching Dr. Cheek work with patients, I had the immediate sense that hypnosis techniques connected mind with body. For me, it was a missing link. Almost instantly I realized that there was more to healing than I had been taught in medical school. The mind-body link revived a major interest in Eastern religions that I had developed in college. At Brown University I had taken a course called "Yoga, Immortality and Freedom" from Kees Bolle, a history-of-religions scholar who had trained under Mircea Eliade, the famous University of Chicago professor and author. From Bolle and Eliade I had become interested in yoga's ability to profoundly affect the body and mind. I discovered that certain mind states achieved in meditation and imagery result in a change in consciousness or understanding that dispels ignorance and results in personal transformation. Meditation takes us to a new level of consciousness, one in which we can feel and understand the world in a different way. The concept of there being two different worlds—the daily world, as opposed to the sacred world—made a great impression on me. With exposure to hypnosis, I began to glimpse the fact that imagery produced physical healing as well as transformation.

After my residency, I joined the Public Health Service to do immunology research at the National Institutes of Health; however, by destiny I was assigned instead to the Hopi Indian Reservation at Keams Canyon, Arizona. There, I was faced with two completely different realities: the spiritual realities of the Hopis and Navahos, who traditionally had deep ties to the Earth and its spirits, and the contrasting realities of pneumonia, infectious diarrhea in infants, and alcoholism in adults. I continued to use my medical training there, practicing allopathic medicine (drugs and surgery) under tremendous time constraints. Because we were understaffed and busy, the average patient visit was four minutes. Moreover, there were no translators for the patients. I would watch the Indians come into our large, sterile hospital and move from one plastic chair to the next as they inched toward their visit with the doctor. At one station they'd be given a chart; at the next they'd have a thermometer stuck in their mouth. Finally they would see the doctor. Then, in only several minutes, they would be given a prescription, often a renewal, for antibiotics or painkillers, or perhaps be sent for an X ray. In time, I found that what I thought I was doing and what my patients thought was happening were two completely different realities. I thought that the medicines I prescribed were helping the Indians physiologically. In fact, my patients incorporated what we were doing into their own belief systems: the public health nurses would report that they often saw the antibiotic tablets we prescribed lined up around the perimeter of Navaho round houses like an energy field. We also were told that Navahos often brought in their very ill babies not to be cured but to die in the hospital, where their spirits would not contaminate their home, or hogan, which would then have to be rebuilt. My time on the reservation was the most difficult and saddest period of my life. I became depressed and did not want to go to work. I felt only emptiness in my job, but I saw all the fullness and beauty of life in the Indians' spiritual world and in the color and openness of the mesas: What I was doing had no personal meaning for me. Practicing the medicine I had been taught did not make me feel good. I felt that something was missing when I only gave people pills and sutured lacerations. My practice lacked the energy of healing that I had gone into medicine to find. At this time in my life I did not know how to practice medicine in a way that would make me feel alive.

After the Indian reservation, we moved to a small seacoast town north of San Francisco, and I stopped practicing medicine in order to reevaluate my life. I did not know where I was headed but I knew that I had to create a more positive reality for myself based on what I loved. The pain and suffering I experienced made me stop and look at my life. I did not have a physical illness; I had a mental or spiritual one. My soul was calling out to be fed. Not knowing what I wanted to do, I intuitively went back to the most enjoyable part of my past and spent a year taking photographs. I loved the country and the seashore, and they made me whole. Nancy and I bought a piece of land with views of the mountains and the ocean and started to build our own house. In a way we were building our own lives; we tried to create a lifestyle that felt good to us. We learned new skills and came face-to-face with our own limitations. I was afraid of heights, so Nancy did all the high work. (If I wanted our house to be completed, I had to resolve any problems and move on with the work.) From house building I learned that you can undertake a huge project about which you know very little and succeed in it. But to do this, you need to reach outside yourself. We had never built anything and didn't even own any tools, so everything was new and exciting. We met Valentino Agnoli, an architect-builder, who designed our house and was willing to start us out on each new phase of the project. He told us that we could act out of love or out of fear. I realized that in order to succeed I needed to have faith in myself and others, to ask questions and take advice, and to seek help when I needed answers. I learned I could create my physical reality from my dreams and images.

Eventually I went back to practicing medicine in the county department of public health. I enjoyed the contact with people there, but simply giving drugs proved once again to be unfulfilling. My ties to healing were still strong. Photographic images lacked a connection to people, and I had not yet figured out how to use images in healing. About this time, 1970, two oil tankers collided under the Golden Gate Bridge, spilling thousands of gallons of crude oil onto the beaches from Santa Cruz to Tomales. The thick, black, tarlike oil covered the beaches, killing the birds and threatening the fragile ecology of the tide pools. Thousands of volunteers came to West Marin to clean up the beaches and wash the birds. Since I was a county health physician and familiar with the area, I was authorized to set up a clinic to take care of the volunteers. Because this clinic was part of a cooperative effort to heal the Earth, it had a different feeling from other medicine I had done. The clinic was held in a marine biology lab next to the rooms where the birds were cleaned. Health workers who were part of the beach cleanup came in and volunteered to help in the clinic. The care spontaneously became personal and loving; it included nontraditional modes such as massage, in addition to the routine trauma care and tetanus shots for injuries.

One of the doctors who came in to volunteer was Irving Oyle, an osteopath who had recently left an internal medicine practice in New York City. When the oil slick cleanup effort ended, Irving and I realized that the need for a clinic still remained. We were excited by the supportive, nontraditional atmosphere of our clinic and decided to set up a clinic of our own. Headlands Clinic opened in the unused manse of a local church. Both Irving and I agreed that we were not interested in practicing the kind of medicine we had formerly done. But in those years we didn't have a clear idea of what we did want to do. The one basic guideline we decided on was that we would let our feelings be our guide and do what felt good to us. This truly was a mysterious decision and process. To create a new type of medicine, we reached back into our past for tools that we had but which we had never consciously used for healing. I had studied immunology, yoga, meditation, hypnosis, and photography; Irving had a background in bodywork, manipulation, and street theater. Like the clinic at the oil slick, Headlands was open to volunteer healers of all types. Irving and I let it be known that we were interested in alternative healing modalities and that we wanted the patient's experience to include them. Out of this came an ongoing philosophical and practical discussion of what health and sickness were. The discussion included both the patients themselves and whatever healers were at the clinic that day. Alternative healers included massage therapists and a psychologist who used autogenic training, a technique involving relaxation and guided imagery. We also worked with Rolling Thunder, an American Indian medicine man; Helen Palmer, a psychic; and Martin Rossman, a physician who was trained in acupuncture. The energy in the clinic was vibrant and alive. Our patients benefited, and it was a learning experience for all of us. The days were full of light; it was like a rebirth.

It was during this time that I became interested in the inner world as a healing space and began to realize increasingly that what I was doing with myself and my patients was deeper and more complex than simple hypnotic relaxation; it actually involved inner journeys. At that time I read Carl Jung's autobiography, *Memories, Dreams, and Reflections,* and was impressed by his descriptions of the figures he met on inner journeys and their tremendous value in his personal growth and healing. One night I had a particularly vivid dream in which I was being chased by disturbing people. I was frightened and worried. But in the dream a quiet voice said to me, "Do you want to get out of this situation?" I said, "Yes," and a voice said, "Come up here." I rose suddenly to a different space of light, quiet, and peace. That morning as I drove to the public health clinic along a beautiful country road in a valley between two hills, I thought that something significant had happened in the dream, but I wasn't quite sure what it was. Then I remembered the voice, and I thought of Jung's descriptions of his inner figures and wondered whether I had met an inner figure in the dream. An inner voice answered, "Yes, you have, and you can talk to me whenever you wish."

Several weeks later a psychologist from UCLA visited Headlands Clinic. He had developed a course based on Silva Mind Control training and offered to teach it to the clinic staff. During the training I learned many interesting guided imagery techniques, including a guided imagery exercise for meeting an inner guide. When I did the exercises, I met the inner voice from my dream again. He said his name was Braxius and he would answer questions that I had about problems in my life and about healing. I have maintained a relationship with Braxius to this day, and I view this relationship as one of the most important parts of my life. I would be missing a crucial part of my life if I could not continue talking to Braxius and the other inner guides I have met.

Gradually the way I practiced medicine changed, as it did for all of the healers in our clinic. I began to use relaxation and guided imagery as major medical tools, along with drugs and referrals to medical specialists. I also began to use inner guides and inner journeys with patients to help them free their inborn abilities to heal themselves. Because education became a major part of my style of practicing medicine, I thought of writing a book to help people heal themselves. With Hal Bennett, a friend who had written a book on education, I wrote *The Well Body Book*, which was published in 1972. It was one of the first self-help medical books and one of the first primers on holistic medicine. In 1975 Nancy and I coauthored *Seeing with the Mind's Eye*, the first major book on guided imagery and healing. Since then I've increasingly devoted my time to teaching people to use guided imagery and inner journeys for healing. I have written eighteen books on self-help medicine, healing, and guided imagery. In my books I seek to empower people, to make them feel better, and to give them tools and skills for healing.

During the past years, my life has changed immensely. For many years I worked with guided imagery and visions with patients with life-threatening illness. I led workshops with Jeanne Achterberg and Frank Lawlis for patients and caregivers, using guided imagery as advanced therapeutics. I concentrated on expanding guided imagery to include visions and spiritual experiences. This made the imagery more powerful and effective. I also shared guided imagery experiences with patients at Commonweal in cancer retreats in Bolinas, California, and learned a great deal from the wonderful people there. I taught a workshop in guided imagery with White Bear Woman at Hollyhock in British Columbia and learned about medicine wheels and healing. I shared my spirit animals with the patients there, and she built a sweat lodge and introduced me to Native American prayer rituals for healing. My interest in shamanic healing has grown and continued to this day.

During this time, I became passionately interested in using art in healing. I started a nonprofit organization, *Art as a Healing Force*, with my sister Linda Samuels to explore how art and healing work together. We held three international invitational conferences that brought together artists and healers, curators and philanthropists, and I met artist healers like Alex Grey, Christiane Corbat, and Vijali Hamilton, who have become dear friends. I started working with writing, art, music, and dance with my patients and realized that art made guided imagery clearer and was a wonderful healing tool. I began to offer art to each patient as part of the healing process.

Then, Nancy, my wife of twenty-six years, was diagnosed with breast cancer. I took care of her for four years. As her death approached, I completely stopped practicing medicine and writing. After a brave healing journey, she died of breast cancer in 1993. After her death, I reexamined my life and decided to start anew. I decided to only do what I loved but realized that my priorities had changed, my intent had sharpened. The spiritual visions around Nancy's death changed me completely. When she died, she became spirit, she became love. She shed her personality and was surrounded by light. In visionary space, she told me that she was giving me the gift of love. She held out her hands, love was in them, and she told me to share her love across the membrane with my patients and the people in my life.

After months of grieving, I slowly started my work anew. I began lecturing, seeing patients and writing, one at a time, to see what I wanted to do. I felt my body with each task. I slowed down and tried to see how, deep inside, each thing I did made me feel. I realized again that patient care grounded me. Now I could see my patients with love—my eyes were different. I was seeing out of the eyes of someone across the membrane who could see with love; Nancy had given me that gift with her death. In addition to my patient care, my lectures became richer and more emotional. I realized that they also connected me to a larger world. Nancy was even present at many lectures after her death. Lecture after lecture there would be one empty chair next to mine. I could see her and feel her presence and hear her voice teaching cancer patients how to live fully in love. I slowly realized that I loved all the things I did, I had done them for important reasons, and I realized this was who I was. Taking my life apart and putting it together with intent, one piece at a time, sharpened my focus and made me clear about who I was and where I wanted to go on my healing journey.

One day, months after Nancy's death, I asked to fall in love. A wonderful woman was given to me and I became a spirit lover. She was a musician and led an organization in art in healing. I wrote love poetry, traveled, and with my lover became more deeply involved in art in healing. Being in love was wonderful, I was seeing out of the eyes of a spirit lover, the world was new, purified. Judgment disappeared, beauty replaced that critical voice within. Art as a Healing Force, the organization I had set up before Nancy's death, was growing. I was now networking programs all over the world that put artists into hospitals with cancer patients. I led several more conferences on art in healing and met more artist healers. I met Mary Rockwood Lane at a conference and visited the Arts in Medicine Program at the University of Florida. Mary and I wrote *Creative Healing* together about how art heals, and she shared her research project "Spirit Body Healing" about art and spirituality. *Spirit Body Healing* became our next book together. It is a book about creativity and spirituality as healing tools. Since then, I have been increasingly involved in creativity and spirituality in health care.

The other great change in my life has come from shamanism. I have taken that part of me and expanded it and let it grow. I have become a healing bear dancer with Native Americans and I work with cancer patients and shamanic healing. The shamanic themes in this book have expanded and grown until they are now a larger part of my life. My book *The Path of the Feather,* and my book *Shaman Wisdom, Shaman Healing,* written with Mary Rockwood Lane, reflect these expanded shamanic interests. I believe that shamanism is a powerful healing modality that heals the soul. It is a gateway to transformation, a magical way of changing the body through the soul. It stimulates spiritual DNA and heals with memories of the ancestors.

My journey is one toward healing with spirit. In the years since I have been a physician, healing the body has been replaced by healing the body, mind, and spirit. I have been privileged to be a pioneer in this body-mind healing process. My journey is a journey to honor patients with love and work with them to heal their souls.

In addition to an ordinary introduction that deals with important inner and outer events in a person's life, I also like to use a more playful, whimsical introduction in which you describe an animal that you are attracted to at this moment, and why. The animal may be a creature that you are simply drawn to or one you have liked for years. It may be a pet, an animal you've seen at the zoo, a wild animal, or even a mythological animal. I have found that animals are powerful symbols, and their spirits are valuable for healing. For thousands of years the symbols of animals have been used by many traditional peoples to confer protection and power.

Here is my animal introduction: Today I see myself as a large black bird with powerful wings, a sharp beak, and strong wings. I can see clearly in the distance and can soar high in the air toward my nest in the faraway mountains. (I love birds, and hawks and turkey buzzards soar and hunt in the area around my house.)

In a workshop, I would now ask the participants to introduce themselves, going around the circle. This is one of the most important and enjoyable parts of a workshop. Each person makes a gift of himself or herself in the introduction. Their strengths are special and help to uplift everyone; their weaknesses make them human and allow us all to grow. When we realize that people still love and value us in spite of our weaknesses or illnesses, we feel validated and strengthened. If we had no weaknesses or problems or illnesses, we'd have no need to change. For many people, this need for change or the desire to grow is what brings them to a workshop. The personal introduction helps people to define both their present situation and their vision. It begins the process of reframing their view of the world to allow change to occur. Often the introduction will spontaneously bring up new insights that define your needs and make you aware of what you really want.

In a book, as opposed to a workshop, your own introduction puts you in the book and provides a step toward becoming actively involved. In thinking of your introduction, you may find it helpful to look at it as if it were a myth, a myth that depicts your path through life with some coherence. Your own myth takes disparate incidents from your past and frames them in a way that is either linear or loosely connected. Your introduction need not encompass all the events in your life nor be strictly chronological—simply include those events or images that seem meaningful to you at this moment. Sometimes people find that the most spontaneous, disparate themes can be the most successful. Your images may be of inner or outer events, of adult or childhood concerns. It is often useful to include both low times and high ones, moments of suffering and of bliss, weaknesses and strengths.

In the introduction, it's also useful to figure out what you want from the book and what your goals are now. If you have an illness, define it and go over its history. Clarify its diagnosis and your feelings about it. Your personal introduction may make you feel uplifted or upset. If you've found it disturbing, go back over it in your mind and concentrate on your personal strengths. Finish with a description of your goals and some positive way of achieving them. Concentrate on the things you love best and your strongest and most powerful times. I know this can be difficult. Throughout the book we will work together to help you increase your power and your confidence in yourself. If you do not feel very strong now, be patient. In the metaphorical part of your introduction, bring to mind an animal. Don't worry about what animal you think of; any animal is fine. Your animal will become a symbol of power and strength that you can use for healing.

To work on your introduction, put the book aside. Rest for a few moments and then frame in your mind what you would say to introduce yourself to a small group of people with whom you would be spending the next several hours or days or a doctor with whom you are learning how to use imagery for physical and mental healing or spiritual healing. After you have taken several minutes to talk about yourself mentally, write down some of the key incidents or themes. Then take a few more minutes to see in your mind's eye an image of an animal. Again, take time to write a description of it. This is the beginning of the work. Your thoughts and images start here and will grow. One woman that I worked with was drawn to the image of a cat during the animal part of her introduction. She was a secretary who liked competitive sports and had great personal strength but was afraid of being vulnerable or out of control. She had cancer of the cervix and did not know what to do. Throughout the rest of the workshop the cat grew and grew and finally was transformed into a huge black panther. For this woman the panther stood for strength, power, and courage. It also had the ability to be gentle and nurturing. The panther combined strength and gentleness. Later, this woman discovered a gentleness within her own strength that she had never realized, which opened up a whole new dimension in her ability to relate to and take care of herself. The gentleness enabled her to deal with her illness with less fear and to take control of the decisions she had to make. These realizations made her more whole and allowed her to use her strength in an area of vulnerability.

Finally I would like to discuss intent and acceptance, trying and letting go. Each person who has an illness faces this dilemma. Healing takes place in the context of two seemingly insoluble paradoxes. The first paradox is the difference between actively initiating changes and letting things happen by themselves. This is a profound paradox that has entered into religion, especially Eastern religions, throughout history. It is really the paradox between free will and fate, or free will and predestination. And it is the dilemma that occurs when people try to meditate and relax but are told that both meditation and relaxation involve goalless activity, or letting go. This paradox is actually a crucial one in healing. I believe healing occurs by itself when images or symbols are released from our inner center soul or spirit and come to awareness in our minds. Our minds then relax and send healing messages to our body. When this happens, our body makes shifts in its immune system without our even being aware of it.

Healing happens by itself, but at the same time, if people do not put themselves in a daydream state, a place of reverie where images and symbols are released to consciousness, causing the immune system to shift, then healing doesn't occur, or occurs more slowly. In a sense, this book will happen to you. The experiences in it, if you are open to them, will occur by themselves. But in a very real sense, preparing ourselves for the change to occur is an active process that takes hard work.

Eastern religions have an ancient way of dealing with this paradox: it involves renouncing the fruits of our work. This means that we do the work almost as an offering, and ideally we view the results without attachment or desire. This attitude frees us from pain and suffering when things do not come out exactly as we might have wished; it encourages the work being done in a beautiful spirit of giving and assumes that good effects will occur. In terms of healing, this view of the world is a gift, because we get a tool that allows us to begin healing work and not worry about the exact effects. In this climate of love, as opposed to fear, the healing occurs by itself. This concept is very important, because people tend to give up when they aren't healed by a certain date or when things don't seem to be going exactly as they'd like. In reality, healing takes time to occur and often takes place when we are not aware of it.

The second paradox is the apparent split between mind and body. It's difficult for all of us to understand how thoughts and images affect or are connected to cancer cells or atherosclerotic plaques in the heart. The explanations of scientists are of much value, but it still seems mysterious how our thoughts affect the outer world. The most radical form of this paradox was faced constantly by Eastern religions. Many of them believed that the outer world was a dream *(maya)* created by mind. A well-known story tries to illustrate this paradox: an Indian man who had achieved high levels of meditation skills felt he could control the outer world. While walking down the road, he saw an elephant approach. He sat down and meditated, and in his mind he pictured the elephant disappearing, since he believed that everything around him was created by his mind. The crowd around screamed at him to get up because he was going to be trampled. The elephant's trainer screamed. Finally, when the elephant was about to step on the meditator, a passerby ran out and pushed him safely aside. Profoundly upset, the man went to his teacher and asked why he had failed. In response, the teacher asked him why he hadn't listened to all the voices from his mind asking him to move.

In terms of healing, there are two ways that I deal with this paradox. The first is to have trust; the second is to follow my feelings. Little in medical science has been proven absolutely. Much of our body's magnificent functioning remains a mystery. Science has given us new studies that detail the effect of relaxation and guided imagery on the cardiovascular and immune systems. We now know that relaxation lowers blood pressure and enhances immune functioning. But the broad effects of the mind on life-threatening illnesses are just beginning to be known. For this reason, using guided imagery is, to some degree, an act of trust. Trust itself is probably an ancient healing tool. Trust in the healer is one of the basic factors responsible for the placebo effect and is likely a necessary part of any healing. Trust is also, by no coincidence, one of the essential attributes underlying the relationship between a spiritual seeker and a teacher. Quite simply, trust frees people to do their work. It dispels doubt, calms, reassures, and relaxes.

The second way of dispelling our fears and uncertainties caused by the mind/body paradox is to follow our feelings. Trust is not developed blindly, without any verification. Relaxing imagery is almost immediately experienced as pleasurable. When we use relaxing or positive imagery, we feel better; our energy is increased, and our worries and anxieties are lessened. This pleasurable release acts as a reward that strengthens our trust. The enjoyment that we get from using imagery relieves pain and suffering and is healing in itself. Finally, we don't really have to solve either of the paradoxes intellectually, because our own personal experience acts as our guide.

When we use guided imagery an alchemical change of consciousness frees our body to heal itself. When we take inner journeys and see inner visions, our psyche is rearranged. Spirit, mind, and body act together: the spirit calms the mind, which allows the body to heal. Parts of the mind are put in place; circuits are created that cause our immune system to change. An Eastern parallel to inner transformation is the dispersion of ignorance. Buddhists believe that human pain and suffering are caused by desire and by mistaking our own personalities for the larger powers that maintain the universe. When people realize that they are not separate from the world around them and that their personality doesn't always control events, ignorance is dispelled and they are transformed. The parallels between spiritual growth and healing are a basic theme of this book. I believe that the path toward healing merges with the path of personal growth. Pain and suffering—either spiritual or physical—result in an urgent need for change. An inner journey is undertaken, and after many adventures, the old personality dies. Then, as a natural process, rebirth occurs, the person is released from suffering, and a new body is created. My goal is for both of us to be different by the end of this book, for change to take place, and for us to grow a new body.

The Discussion

The first exercise of the book is a short inner journey designed to introduce you to the feeling of guided imagery. You have already done this in the brief exercise, and you do it all the time when you are daydreaming. But if this type of structured exercise is new to you, you need not be nervous about it. I've done these exercises with thousands of people from all walks of life, and there is nothing to worry about. People who have done the exercises from written material do so in one of two basic ways. One is to go through the exercise slowly as you read it. The other way is to do the exercises after you have read them through, which is preferable. To do this, read the exercise over several times, until you have the general idea of it in your mind. Then sit or lie down in a comfortable position in a place where you will not be disturbed for a half hour or so. Close your eyes and repeat the instructions to yourself. Do not worry about remembering the words exactly; just allow the basic meaning of the instructions to come through. If new, creative ideas arise as you're doing the exercise, feel free to incorporate them. Your own ideas are as important as mine. Start with my ideas and let your own emerge. Allow the experience to take place slowly; give yourself plenty of time to see, feel, hear, smell, and touch. Linger in those parts of your inner journey that are enjoyable, and leave those parts that make you uncomfortable. If extraneous thoughts come into your mind while you're doing the exercises, do not be concerned. This is common. Once you realize you have gotten sidetracked, simply come back to the exercise. The first time you do an exercise like this from memory, it may be difficult and even perplexing. However, with practice, you will find that this is the best way to work, because you become the author of the exercise yourself: you supply the language and images that are the most meaningful to you, that have the richest personal associations. The power of all imagery comes from inside you, and your unconscious knows the most about what will work for you.

There are several other ways to use the exercises in this book. You can make your own tapes by reading the exercises into a tape recorder. Read them slowly, and leave pauses so that images can arise. Your own voice on a tape is very effective. Another way to use the exercises is to have someone read them to you while you sit or lie in a comfortable position. If you wish, you can play peaceful music in the background while you do the exercises. For many people, such music helps them to relax and image.[1]

People who do this exercise for the first time have many different reactions. Most people say the exercise feels very relaxing and calming. Some people enjoy it so much they don't want to return to their everyday world and often lie there relaxing and daydreaming after they have done the exercise. One man, a professional soccer player, came up to me after the first exercise and told me that he was totally surprised to find himself in tears throughout the whole exercise. Apparently he had discovered a new and soft place inside himself. Enjoy the exercise, drift with it, and let the images carry you. Don't worry about doing it right; don't worry if your mind wanders and you think of other things. Don't worry if it feels strange at first. All these reactions are normal. We all need more time to dream.

The Exercises

Exercise 1—Starting on the Path.

Find a comfortable space where you will not be disturbed. Sit or lie down with your legs uncrossed, your arms at your sides or resting on your abdomen. Loosen any tight or constricting clothing. Close your eyes. Begin by inhaling slowly and deeply through your nostrils. Let the breath out through your nose slowly and completely. Continue breathing in this manner, allowing your abdomen to rise as you inhale and fall as you exhale. As you breathe allow yourself to relax.

Now imagine that your feet are touching the ground on a path in the country. The path is made of dirt and is well trodden. On each side of the path are trees. It's a late summer afternoon. Follow the path, feeling the ground under your feet as you walk. The path leads slightly downward, so walking is easy. Smell the freshness of the air and feel its balminess against your skin as you walk. You can hear your feet make gentle contact with the ground and see the path under your feet. As you walk, allow your troubles and cares to slip away. Imagine that each problem you are worried about comes off you and falls to the ground. You can simply let your cares drop off, or you can deliberately put them in a box, label them, and place them on the ground alongside the path. The cares you leave behind may be concerns about your family, your work, or an illness. As you leave your cares behind, you will feel yourself become lighter and your walking will be easier and more upright. You will have more energy and feel more peaceful.

Now you see ahead of you an unusual circle of pine trees. The circle is about twenty feet in diameter, and the trees are planted about two feet apart. The trees are very tall and old. The path leads into the circle between two trees. Walk into the circle and stop in the center. Feel the awesome quiet created by this magical circle. Inhale the aromatic pine smell, feel the soft cushion of pine needles under your feet, and notice the delicate lighting created by the branches. Let the energy from the trees flow into your body. Let the healing energy of nature come up into the trees and into you. Feel the energy as buzzing or tingling. As the energy flows into you, you can imagine any remaining worries slipping away. Now imagine a warm, gentle rain falling into the center of the circle, washing over you and making you feel cleansed and more alive. Let the water drip down your body and wash away tension, illness, and cares. When the rain stops, the sun shines through the trees and almost instantly dries you off.

Follow the path as it leads out the other side of the circle. The path now slopes gently upward. As it climbs, the terrain becomes drier and the ground harder. As you climb, you feel a sense of renewed energy from the pine tree clearing, and your legs feel warm and strong. The air smells sharper and lighter. Off to your left you can see the sun start to dip toward the horizon. The path finally leads through a small rural village, made up of a few stucco houses that lie some distance off the path to either side. Some people have come to the side of the path to wish you well on your journey. They smile, call words of encouragement, and wave at you. Several people even scatter flower petals on the path as you walk by. Some of the people may be familiar to you; you may notice friends, loved ones, or teachers wishing you on.

Leave the village behind you and continue climbing the gentle path. Now the path becomes a little steeper and begins to ascend the right side of a rocky gorge. As it climbs, you can hear a stream gurgling down in the gorge. Finally you come to a beautiful wooden bridge that spans the shallow gorge. The bridge is about fifty feet long and arches slightly. It is made of solid, smooth, well-worn planks that lie crosswise to the bridge. The bridge has a stout railing on either side. Start walking across the bridge. Hear the hollow echo as your feet hit the planks. With each footfall you become more relaxed and full of energy. As you listen to the burbling of the stream, let any remaining cares and worries you might have float away with the stream.

As you look across the bridge, you realize that the other

side is a completely different terrain. As you get closer to it, you feel larger, stronger, and more powerful. The energy in you becomes more intense and your senses become clearer. Across the bridge is a dirt path across a grass-covered plain. The ground here is moister and softer, but the air is still high and clear. After a time, you come to a striking meadow that is fairly large. It is now dusk, and the brightest stars can be seen faintly in the darkening sky. The meadow is about a hundred yards across and has an unusual rectangular shape bordered by clumps of trees. In the center of the meadow is a slight bowl-shaped depression. Far off in the distance, past each corner of the meadow, you can see one of four tall, snow-covered mountains. Directly above the meadow is a group of bright stars.

Looking around, you can see that many other people are coming to the meadow on different paths, and begin to sit in a large circle in the center of the meadow. Find your place in the circle and sit down. Look around the circle and notice friends and loved ones, healers and helpers. Imagine that about a hundred feet above the center of the circle is a point of energy. Imagine that the point emits a white light that has a slight bluish tinge. The light coming from the ball spreads out to form a cone over the people. Feel the energy from the ball flow into your body. The energy is soft, healing, and relaxing. Now stand up and look at the cone. You will see a shadowlike shape on the cone in front of you. It looks something like the indentation that people make when they lie on the sand at the beach. Lean forward until your body fits perfectly in the indentation; the cone will support you. The cone is pure energy—your head will be supported without interfering with your breathing. Allow yourself to rest in the indentation, and feel the energy flowing from the top of the cone, through your body, and down into the ground. Allow all pain, tension, and illness to flow out of your body and into the ground. Let the energy make you feel vibrant and whole. Stay there as long as you wish.

To return, you will retrace your steps. Stand up and leave the meadow. Follow the familiar path back to the bridge and hear your footsteps echo again on the wooden planks. Walk back on the same path past the little village and go upward to the pine tree circle. This time follow a path around the circle of trees to the right. It joins the old path past the trees. Now follow that path back upward to where you started.

When you wish to return to your everyday state, gently move your feet and count slowly from one to three. You will return to your everyday state relaxed, comfortable, and full of energy. Your body will feel as if it is in a comfortable, healing space. Each time you do this exercise you will relax more deeply and more easily. The feelings of relaxation will deepen, and the whole exercise will become more and more pleasurable.

Rest a moment and enjoy the feelings from the exercise. How did the exercise make you feel? As you will realize, the answer to this question is not simple. The goal of this first exercise is direct experience. So for now, just try to identify or remember the feelings evoked by the exercise and the difference between your thoughts during the exercise and your everyday thoughts. After this first exercise, many people continue resting and do not want to get up. The relaxation they feel is much deeper than they are used to and is intensely pleasurable. Many people can actually feel the ground under their feet as they imagine walking, and experience intense feelings of purification during the pine tree shower. Some people aren't aware of imagery but simply experience lightness and a restful feeling during the exercise. Afterward, people who are unfamiliar with guided imagery may be frustrated by not having intense feelings during the exercise. They will find that the specific exercises in the next chapter will help make them more aware of their imagery. One man, a psychologist, said that although he was not really aware of any specific imagery, he had never relaxed as deeply in his life. He felt that his body was floating and tingling and that he was in a half-awake state. He said he felt as if the exercise was a massage from within, as if an external force was filling him with energy. He finished the exercise with feelings of being connected to the universe.

If you wish, you can keep a notebook to describe the imagery experiences that you have. You may also find it relevant to write down dreams, visions, and experiences that you have concurrently. In workshops I also advise people to spend time outdoors in nature between exercises. This helps to connect them to the source of life and allows the Earth to heal them. Immerse yourself in nature as much as the place you live in permits. See the world around you as sacred. Specific problems in relaxing or imaging will be discussed at the end of the next chapter. In this first exercise, the experience itself was key. I remind you that during an exercise such as this, real physiological changes take place within your body. As you relax, your heartbeat slows, your blood pressure drops, and your breathing slows. Your immune system is activated and healing neurotransmitters are released in your brain. The healing is real. You've already started; it's easy and simple.

2

THE VEHICLE:
REVERIE STATES

By changing our consciousness, we can promote healing. Everyone is capable of doing this. I have worked with men and women from varied backgrounds—differing races, economic groups, professions, and ages. I enjoy working with people because of the energy exchanged in the experience, but even more important, I value the healing and growth that I see. When people come to me depressed and anxious, and leave feeling positive and full of joy, it is a great pleasure. After this work, people feel different; they feel more connected, reassured, and at peace. Helping people to travel inward is one of the most enjoyable things I do.

Healing comes from the inner world. Understanding this process is crucial because it allows us to heal ourselves. More precisely, physical healing occurs at the interface where inner and outer join. Healing is enhanced when we go within, listen to our inner world, trust the information, and let it empower us. Now that we have started traveling inward, we can begin to work more purposefully. The feelings that you had in the first exercises can be deepened and tuned to promote healing.

We enter our inner world through an imaginary journey, and the vehicle for that journey is a state of consciousness called the reverie state. The reverie state involves feelings of relaxation and dreaminess similar to a pleasurable daydream. It is a time of letting go of the troubles of the outer world, relaxing, and letting a greater force direct us. For all of recorded history, people have realized that the reverie state was a doorway to healing as well as to spiritual enlightenment. But it's only in recent years that physicians have worked in an organized way to make use of this knowledge. I will teach you to use the reverie state to enhance your own healing.

One of the basic concepts of medicine is that our body heals itself. The body has a powerful immune system that is capable of destroying viruses, bacteria, and cancer cells, and its remarkable healing mechanisms can clot blood, mend broken bones, dissolve plaques from coronary arteries, and regenerate healthy tissue. The body routinely dissolves and replaces sick, injured, and old cells with healthy new ones. This process is crucial to our life, yet it has been studied very little by modern medicine. In fact, research on healing mechanisms does not even appear in medical textbooks, while information about the immune system has only begun to appear within the last twenty years, under the impetus of research on the newly understood immune system diseases. When a person has surgery, the doctor sews the tissues together, but it is the body that heals. After a person is injured, the body heals itself. After most infections the body heals itself. Not all cancer cells grow into tumors; the body destroys most of them. Drugs and surgery help the body heal but would be ineffective without the body's own healing powers.

In the past, the immune system of our body was not thought to be under our conscious control, nor did we understand what makes it function more or less effectively. Now we know that many body functions such as breathing and heartbeat are affected by our thoughts and perceptions. Medical researchers are now beginning to understand that thoughts and perceptions also affect our immune system and our ability to heal. Moreover, many researchers have come to believe that our basic philosophical outlook has a profound effect on how well or poorly our immune system works. It is now accepted that some mental attitudes are healing and others are not. Specific images cause physiological changes in blood flow and immune function. If the images are of a certain type, healing is enhanced. Thus, we can help our body heal by changing our consciousness.

The characteristics of the reverie state coincide with those qualities that produce health; this occurrence is not accidental. In fact, I believe that the reverie state evolved as the body's mechanism to heal itself and to make itself whole. When crucial paradoxes are resolved, it's almost as if, in a strange way, the body enters a realm that, for lack of understanding, we call miraculous. Knowledge of the miraculous side of healing gives us tremendous power. When we discover we can help heal ourselves, we grow stronger and begin to heal. Each characteristic of the reverie state facilitates this effect.

In this chapter we will discuss the reverie state and how it helps heal the body. To understand the reverie state, we must first analyze our thought processes. For reasons that are not fully understood, people view their thought processes as being different for inner and outer worlds. This feeling may be due to the specialization between right and left brain. The outer world consists of physical events that take place in time and space; it involves getting information from our senses and acting on that information. A typical example of an outer world activity is walking. Our senses are alert, and our body moves in response to what we perceive in the outer world. By comparison, in the inner world the action takes place in our mind. We turn away from the world of our senses and go to a reality that exists inside our mind. Our eyes are closed, our senses are dampened, and we move only in our mind.

Not all time spent in the inner world is time spent in the reverie state. All of us know that we spend a lot of time thinking, worrying, planning, and problem solving in relation to our activities in the outer world. When we leave the outer world, go into our minds, and purposefully picture scenes or experience an inner dialogue, we enter the reverie state, which has a different feeling from the outer world. This difference in feeling is a crucial distinction.

For thousands of years people have attempted to define or clarify the different states, or levels, of consciousness. Neither ancient nor modern scholars have solved the puzzle. Common terms used to describe the reverie state are "altered state of consciousness," "shamanic state of consciousness," "meditational state," "mystical and now guided imagery state," "religious feeling of awe or ecstasy," "trance state." Although they are difficult to define scientifically, these levels of consciousness are so universally a part of humanity's experience through the ages that their reality cannot be denied. The single factor common to all of them is that they feel different from everyday consciousness. People's thinking is altered when they are in a reverie state. Interestingly, these levels of consciousness have always been credited with tremendous power, in that they were universally believed to affect physical reality. For that reason, historically they have been the doorway to healing and to the control of the outer world. They have also been a gateway to spiritual growth and mystical enlightenment in many religions of the world. We can learn much from the extreme importance credited to reverie states and from the techniques developed by experts through thousands of years of trial and error. It is time that we make use of this knowledge. The reason that most people find it so easy to work in the reverie state is that intuitively they sense it is right. The reverie state is our birthright; we evolved to experience reverie.

Most events in life involve a combination of different states of consciousness. For example, when we are driving, we can be in the awake state, paying attention to our senses, and simultaneously in an altered state in which we daydream. Athletes, during peak performances, can enter a state in which inner and outer become one and their actions seemingly take place by themselves. This state is much like the one in which healing takes place. The common factor is a feeling of oneness with the universe, calmness, and peace. Certain characteristics of the reverie state make it useful for healing and give it power. Here we will discuss them briefly, but as the book unfolds, their depth and complexity will become more apparent. The reverie state is an experience that is felt, not a theory. It is most commonly described as being like a daydream. When you concentrate on an inner rather than an outer image, you are one-minded and not aware of your surroundings.

The exercise that you did at the end of the last chapter was an experience in the reverie state. For some of you the experience may not have been that involving, but the feelings you had were true examples of the reverie state. As you read the subsequent description of the reverie state, try to relate this information to the experiences you just had. See how many of the characteristics of the reverie state you experienced. Because it was a beginning experience, your feelings probably were not as concentrated or dramatic as what I will describe, but they are important. I'm going over this material in detail to help you realize what deeper or more involved reverie states feel like. Many of the sensations are subtle and difficult to keep hold of when you return to your everyday consciousness.

First, reverie alters the way we see the world; it radically affects our sense of time and space. The more profound the reverie experience (i.e., the "deeper" it is), the more that time and space, as we know them in the outer world, tend to disappear. As time and space telescope into a single point or expand into infinity, we come to exist completely in a limitless here and now. Because the reverie state is an immediate state, there is no past or future, no distance. To conceive of the reverie state, one has only to think of a dream. The dreamer has no past or future, and space is discontinuous. When time and space evaporate, so do the laws of physics. Gravity is gone; the solidity of physical bodies disappears; you can even be in more than one place at a time. From a healing standpoint, being here and now in the reverie state not only relieves worries, it confers magical powers, magical in that they do not have to obey the laws of time and space. The reverie state allows situations to be rehearsed that could not take place in the physical world, and part of the mind clearly obeys the laws of the reverie state and sends healing messages to the body. Myth and symbol are without time and space, and creation legends are timeless in that they are still occurring. We create our reality anew every moment.

Along with the changes in time and space that take place in the reverie state come a change in understanding. There is a decrease in logical thinking, in thinking that deals with cause and effect, and an increase in immediate, feeling-oriented thinking. Because the reverie space isn't tied to simple physical laws, much more complex understandings can be grasped. One is the coexistence of opposites, or paradoxes, which has previously been discussed. This concept is extremely useful in healing, involving the mind-body paradox and the paradox of acting and letting go at the same time. Because the reverie state can bridge these paradoxes, it frees our body to heal itself.

Another characteristic of the reverie state is a sense of loss of control. In a strange way, this sense or feeling is also paradoxical. The personality, or ego, feels as if it's losing control, but in fact the individual is gaining greater control by merging the personality's aims with those of a force that is greater than the ego. People view that force as their true Self, as Nature, or as a spiritual force. It is this loss of ego and merging with a greater force that shamans and spiritual healers utilize for healing.

The experience of the inner world changes our worldview in ways that are both subtle and profound. First, it gives people a sense that they understand the world around them. This feeling imparts a sense of illumination, of sudden understanding, thereby making the unclear clear. Although these realizations feel very deep to the person who is experiencing them, they are difficult to put into words. Because the experiences are too complex and deep to express in words, they have a sense of mystery and excitement. This aspect of the unknown, coupled with a sense of seeking answers to the most profound questions, reawakens people's interest in living and renews their sense of purpose. These feelings are revitalizing. An intense desire to live is also associated with increased health. After inner journeys, people commonly have feelings of rejuvenation or rebirth. They feel cleansed, as if they were starting anew, and they experience spontaneous feelings of new hope. One woman that I worked with was depressed and worried about her family. During a guided imagery exercise, she found herself in a cave talking to Mother Earth, whose voice told her to "let go" and allow her children to be themselves. She finished the exercise with a tremendous feeling of calmness and a positive vision of her family's future. A very simple thought had great power for her when it came from within a reverie state.

Because inner experiences are difficult to describe in words, people often have trouble retaining a sense of their experience when they are not in the inner world. As time passes in the outer world, the insights of the inner world are often forgotten. There is a sense of amnesia, somewhat like waking up from a dream. Myths and symbols are a way of giving form to this type of inner understanding that transcends the rational. Profound feelings of understanding are transformative in themselves. People are comfortable when they comprehend the world around them; they feel at home. Events become understandable and predictable. In studies, such feelings have been shown to be associated with good health, as we shall see in the next chapter.

Along with a change in meaning and worldview, there comes a change in feeling. People have powerful emotional experiences in the inner world. Intense feelings of joy and delight go along with feelings of profound understanding. These emotions are spontaneous and direct. Because they do not tend to be colored by personality, they have the sharpness of childhood feelings. These emotions span a wide range from ecstasy to fear and relate directly to whatever the person is experiencing. The reverie state is also a doorway to the darkness. Each of us has feelings of fear, anger, pain, loss, and alienation that can emerge in inner visions. As these feelings surface, deep healing occurs. Often feelings of intense wellbeing, joy, and love accompany inner experiences that are beautiful or universal. One of the goals of inner journeys is to have experiences in a place of peace where deep, positive emotions are freed.

Another characteristic of inner space is enhanced suggestibility. People on inner journeys are in a receptive place to receive suggestions from trusted figures. Suggestions from doctors, psychologists, hypnotists, and shamans, as well as inner guides, can exert a profound influence on a person in the inner world. Likewise, intuitive feelings from the inner center play a greater role in changes that come from the inner world. The value of this increased suggestibility for healing is obvious. People are more likely to undertake the kind of work necessary to heal if they are open and receptive to positive suggestions.

The inner world changes our perception of our body image. This change is so deep and confusing—and fascinating—that it intrigues everyone who works with the inner world. Even in an imagery state that is not very deep, people can notice that they are not aware of their body in the normal way. In the everyday world people orient themselves through their sense organs: they are always aware of gravity, of pressures on their body; they feel equilibrium; they hear sounds that orient them spatially; they see things around them that increase their sense of an outer world. Generally, people feel as if their consciousness lies in that part of their body that is most active at any given moment. This is especially important in reference to pain or illness. The painful or ill area of the body holds people's attention, but when people are in the inner world, their consciousness is not in their physical body. If they're imagining walking down a path, their real body is not feeling the ground and smelling the air; an imaginary body is doing this. While people are experiencing an inner journey, their real body is lying down or sitting in a chair. During an inner journey, people feel as if their real body is functioning automatically, taking care of itself, while their consciousness is in their imaginary body. In a real feeling sense, their consciousness is out of their physical body. When most people initially enter the reverie state, during a relaxation exercise, for example, their consciousness feels as if it is in or very near their physical body. But when they relax more deeply or image a scene such as walking down a path, their consciousness feels as if it is floating outside them or in the body that they are imagining. This feeling ranges from mild to profound and can be associated with feelings of expansion of consciousness, expansion of space, and a sense of oneness. The sense of oneness includes the dissolution of physical boundaries and the merging of all things.

During a relaxation experience or an experience in which people are picturing a part of their body, they experience sensations in their physical body as well as in their imaginary body. Generally these sensations are described as tingling, buzzing, pulsing, numbness, lightness, or heaviness. These feelings have been shown to be associated with verifiable physiological changes such as changes in blood flow, a reduction in muscle tension, and a decrease in pain sensations. There are definitely links between mental images and changes in body physiology, including changes in the immune system. The physical body cannot distinguish between real and imagined perceptions, and it responds similarly to both.

Often people's consciousness jumps back and forth between their imaginary body in the inner world and their real body in the outer world. In fact, this jumping back and forth, grounding and going out, is both common and useful in beginning imagery. It helps to give people a sense of control, even as they are letting go of control. Only in deeper trance states do people lose track of their physical body and immediate surroundings for more than a brief period. During light trance states, a part of the person always knows where he or she is. This does not stop a person from experiencing the value of the exercise.

The feeling of being in an imaginary body, outside one's physical body, is an extremely valuable one for healing. First, by taking a person's consciousness out of the body, it allows the body to function under the direction of the inner self. When the body works automatically, blood flow and immune responses aren't impaired by tension, and healing mechanisms function optimally. Second, it allows people to work on their body with more objectivity and less fear. When people envision an imaginary body, they can see problems and work on them with less concern. The objectivity, or distance, takes away fear and increases power. Finally, when people feel as if they're outside of their body, they're not as bothered, emotionally or physically, by pain and illness. When people imagine that they are somewhere else, with practice they can leave pain behind with their physical body. One of the best pain-control methods involves having people imagine that they are rising out of their body and drifting elsewhere. This technique was perfected by hypnotherapists and is used for anesthesia. People can even imagine looking down on their body or looking at it from another room. This dissociation changes people's perception of pain and brings comfort. It is similar to watching television and concentrating so completely on the show that one's attention is distracted from a pain.

There is no doubt in the minds of physicians and psychologists who work with guided imagery that images can affect the physiology of the body and cause healing. Those people who have used guided imagery to heal their own illnesses have an experiential knowledge of how imagery affects the body. For many years, mind-body researchers have been working on a scientific model to describe the relationship between mental states and healing. This model is essential for several reasons. First, a very detailed model that can be verified helps to incorporate the concept into mainstream medicine. Second, a model helps people who are starting with guided imagery to have greater trust in and understanding of imagery's power until they have firsthand experience of it. Last, the more we know about guided imagery, the more we are able to distinguish the most important aspects of imagery work and thus make the techniques increasingly effective.

Currently the field of mind-body medicine is a rapidly expanding, exciting subject of research and practice. In past years, thousands of papers have been written concerning the effects of mind states on illness.[1] For a person who's interested in using the techniques immediately, it's very useful to have a basic physiological understanding of how guided imagery works and what direction the most current research is taking. Although the model is technical, it is interesting and understandable.

The first major concept is that mind and body are interconnected. What we call consciousness or thought is somehow involved with the firing of neurons in our brain, and the brain is connected to the rest of the body, including the hormonal and immune systems, via the spinal cord and peripheral nerves. The nervous system is divided into two parts, central and peripheral. The *central nervous system*, which consists of the brain and spinal cord, is composed of trillions of nerve cells that are connected and interconnected into circuits, or loops. The brain itself is made up of the *forebrain, midbrain,* and *hindbrain.* The forebrain is further separated into two areas, one of which contains the cerebral cortex and limbic system, while the other contains the thalamus, hypothalamus, and pituitary gland. The *peripheral nervous system* is made up of the *somatic nervous system,* which delivers nerve impulses to and from the muscles and sensory receptors, and the *autonomic nervous system,* which innervates the heart, lungs, intestines, and other internal organs. The autonomic nervous system is responsible for maintaining the body's internal equilibrium, including heart rate, respiratory rate, digestion, hormonal production and balance, electrolyte balance, and so on. When I went to medical school, I was taught that these functions were automatic, but now it is known that we have some control over these homeostatic, or self-regulating, mechanisms. Since the autonomic nervous system controls the actual chemical balances of the body, it is obviously the key system in connecting the mind to the body.

The autonomic nervous system is divided into two parts: the sympathetic and the parasympathetic. The autonomic nervous system affects the body immediately via nerves that innervate the body's organs and blood vessels, and over a longer period of time via the stress hormones of the adrenal gland (e.g., adrenaline). The *sympathetic nervous system* is basically concerned with getting the body ready for action in the outside world. People feel the effects on their sympathetic nervous system whenever they are in a situation of danger or anxiety. The heart beats faster, blood pressure rises, respiration increases, sugar is released from the liver for quick action, and blood is directed away from the digestive system to the voluntary muscles. This general reaction, in which a person experiences a pounding heart and knots in the stomach, is referred to as the *fight-or-flight reaction*. Prolonged anxiety, which keeps the body in a constant state of sympathetic arousal, literally wears the body down and makes it more susceptible to all types of illness. The *parasympathetic nervous system*, in contrast, takes over when the body is relaxed and peaceful. It creates balance, homeostasis, and healing. It slows the heart rate and respiratory rate, drops the blood pressure, and directs blood to the digestive organs. A useful simplification to keep in mind is that one part of the nervous system reacts to the body's perception of danger through action in the outer world, and the other part of the nervous system reacts to the body's perceptions of peace by balancing the body in the inner world. Healing illness is simply a natural extension of the body's homeostatic mechanisms.

The cerebral cortex is made up of two hemispheres connected by a large bundle of nerve fibers. Researchers have found that the left side of the brain has specialized to some degree in language processing, analysis, and linear thinking. The right hemisphere is responsible for storage and retrieval of images and for nonverbal thought. The right hemisphere seems to deal more with body image, processing emotional information, and reacting to stress. The right hemisphere is richly connected with the *limbic system,* which mediates our emotions and is involved with feelings of pleasure, pain, and anger. Another useful simplification is to say that the left hemisphere helps control our reactions to the external world, through language and conscious body movements, while the right hemisphere communicates with the internal world of images and emotions. Images are most likely stored in the anterior aspect of the frontal lobes of the right hemisphere. Below the limbic system is the *hypothalamus,* which regulates the body chemistry and the immune system, both directly and through its connections to the master gland, the *pituitary.* The pituitary regulates metabolism through the adrenal glands and the thyroid, as well as the ovaries and testes.

To summarize the complex connection between the mind and the body, we might say that when a person has a perception, either from the outer or inner world, neurons fire in the cerebral cortex and images form in the anterior right brain, which in turn stimulates the limbic system and then the hypothalamus and pituitary gland. Depending upon whether the person's perception is interpreted as peaceful or upsetting, the parasympathetic or sympathetic nervous system will be activated, and that reaction will be sustained by the hormones of the adrenals. The hormones and nerve cells that are stimulated will cause changes in literally every cell in the body.

Recently, scientists have begun to piece together a second major aspect of the way mental processes affect the body. This theory has developed along with the field of immunology, which is the study of how the body defends itself against bacteria, viruses, and cancer cells. Central to this work is the concept that thoughts in the mind cause activity of the immune system to increase or decrease. There are intricate interactions between the brain, the central nervous system, and the immune system. This knowledge has given birth to a whole new field, *psychoneuroimmunology* (PNI). PNI developed from the research of Dr. Robert Ader, who showed that the immune system actually has the ability to "learn"—not just to recognize a foreign substance and make anti-bodies, but to be conditioned to react automatically to life events. In one study rats were given an immunosuppressive agent that lowered the ability of their immune system to function. At the same time they were given a sweetening agent. Later, just the sweetening agent alone would produce a decrease in immune function. This reaction represents classical Pavlovian conditioning. The fact that this conditioning effect takes place has far-reaching ramifications. In this case, the perception of sweetness came to trigger a whole set of physiological responses by which the brain suppressed the immune system. The mind, rather than an external agent, was then controlling the immune system.

Based on the conditioning experiments of Ader, we can postu-late that when people experience emotions or life events that have been associated with illness in the past, their immune system can learn to suppress itself. Initially, scientists did not understand how this could occur, but now they've worked out several pathways. First, during the early 1980s doctors actually discovered nerve end-ings in the immune organs such as the thymus, lymph nodes, spleen, and bone marrow. The presence of these nerves suggests a complex communicating system between the brain and the immune system. Second, researchers have found autonomic nerve fibers in the immune tissues of the tonsils, appendix, and the Peyer's patches of the intestine. Finally, and possibly most impor-tant, the immune system's white blood cells, including lympho-cytes, monocytes, and macrophages, have been shown to respond to chemical messengers from the central nervous system. The white blood cells have on their surface receptors that bind complex mol-ecules such as hormones, neurotransmitters, and neuropeptides.

Neuropeptides, compounds that are produced by the brain, are natural opiates or painkillers. They have been termed *endor-phins*. They are found in high concentrations in the limbic system and other areas known to be involved in pain transmission and processing of emotions. The endorphins have been credited with increased pain tolerance during childbirth and acts of heroism. It has been postulated that they are responsible for pain relief achieved with placebos. In other words, they are self-produced pain relievers. Endorphins are produced in response to reverie states, pleasurable states, exercise, and sweets. In addition to being pain relieving, the endorphins also produce euphoria. Thus, imagining pleasurable states seems to stimulate the limbic system in the brain to produce neuropeptides, which are picked up by immune cells. The neuropeptides then affect the immune cells' activities—their ability to move, to learn, and, most interestingly, to produce their own neuropeptides, which subsequently are picked up by receptors in the brain. They also increase the immune cells' ability to replicate and to attack cancer cells. Thus the immune system can talk to the brain, and the brain to the immune system. This interaction is registered in the limbic system and felt by the person as emotion, as feelings of well-being, in particular joy, hope, and love.

There are now numerous studies that indicate that these mechanisms work to heal illness. The studies basically fall into two groups. The first group links perceptions of life experiences with health or illness and illustrates how depression, loneliness, and hopelessness make illness more likely. The importance of this type of study is that it demonstrates that mental states affect health. In the next chapter we'll discuss in greater detail the studies dealing with attitude. The second group of studies relates life experiences to changes in physiology. These studies help to prove the model that mental states act on the nervous system and the immune system. Briefly, researchers have found that prolonged stress basically causes a decrease in immune function. Specifically, it causes a decrease in lymphocyte proliferation, antibody production, natural killer cell activity, and helper T cell activity. Bereavement has also been shown to result in lowered lymphocyte production, while relaxation and imagery have been shown to increase natural killer cell activity and antibody levels. In particular, studies in which people visualized white blood cells attacking germs demonstrated an increase in natural killer cell activity. All of these studies indicate that stress can cause illness by lowering immune function, and more important, that people can learn to voluntarily enhance immune response through reverie states.

These scientific studies are very useful in that they translate the mysterious link between guided imagery and health into examples that we can readily comprehend and have faith in. But there is no question that the "real" or full answers explaining mind-body interactions have yet to be figured out and, in fact, may never be understood. However, we may be able to "know" these things in a nonintellectual sense when we go inside our minds and become one with a power greater than ourselves.

Many of us working in guided imagery have used simplified models to help people understand how images affect the body. Perhaps the most basic is the concept that our body cannot tell a mental image from a physical event. This is illustrated in the East Indian parable about a man who sees a snake in the road and experiences all the sensations of terror: his heartbeat speeds up, his palms become sweaty, and he gets butterflies in his stomach. After his initial fright, the man suddenly realizes that the object of his terror is not a snake at all but a rope lying coiled in the road. At this point he breathes a sigh of relief and relaxes. His heart rate drops, his breathing slows, and his stomach returns to normal. The psychiatrist Carl Jung called this way of looking at the world *psychic reality,* that is to say, what the mind thinks is real *is* real to a person, whether or not there is a physical manifestation of this reality. In this way, ghosts and spirits are real in that they make a person fearful or powerful, whether or not scientists can prove their existence. Obviously, the more deeply people go into the reverie state or the more intensely they experience imagery, the more "real" the psychic reality seems and the more the body's physiology changes in response.

Edmund Jacobsen, the renowned physiologist, demonstrated extensively that when people imagine body movements, the motor nerves in these areas actually fire and the muscle fibers contract. These movements, called micromovements, can be very subtle, but even if they are not visible to the eye, they can be picked up by electromyographic machines. This response is remarkable in itself, but even more interesting is the fact that the body builds nerve circuits, that is, it "learns," based on imagery exercises that result in micromovements. This learning is the basis of the imagery exercises that athletes use to improve their performance. When they picture successful completion of an activity, their performance actually improves. The micromovements improve the athletes' performance as they increase the athletes' confidence in their ability to perform.

Imagery has also been shown to have immediate physiological effects on body systems other than the muscles. It directly affects the gastrointestinal tract, the cardiovascular system, the endocrine system, and even the skin. It affects blood flow, blood glucose levels, and energy mobilization, and as we've mentioned, it affects the immune system. *Autogenic training,* a German system of imagery and relaxation that was developed in the 1930s, has produced thousands of articles showing how imagery affects virtually every organ in the body; there is even X-ray verification of its effects on bowel motility. Perhaps the most remarkable imagery work is a group of studies by Dr. Howard Hall, a psychologist who demonstrated that when people pictured their white blood cells increasing in number, the blood cells increased. Early biofeedback work even demonstrated that people could actually get one particular nerve cell to fire. Finally, Drs. Wayne Smith and John Schneider did an experiment in which they had volunteers imagine that one type of white blood cell, the *neutrophil,* left the bloodstream to fight germs inside the cells of organs. Remarkably, they found that neutrophil blood levels dropped, but not the levels of other white blood cells. Thus research indicates that not only does the mind control the body to a much greater degree than we ever believed, but it does so rather precisely. Guided imagery has been shown to affect coping, life attitudes, immune function, quality of life, and emotional well-being after breast cancer. In an important study at the University of Texas Center for Alternative Medicine Research in Cancer at the University of Texas Health Science Center, Houston, Texas, Mary Ann Richardson assigned women who completed treatment for primary breast cancer to standard care or a six-week support or imagery program. All of the women's immune systems were enhanced, their antibodies (interferon-gamma) increased, and their stress indicators (neopterin) decreased. Their quality of life improved. The research demonstrated that compared with standard care, both support and imagery improved coping skills, attitudes, perception of support, and tended to enhance meaning in the woman's life. When comparing imagery with support, imagery participants tended to have less stress, increased vigor, and improved functional and social quality of life. This study indicates that guided imagery and support are primary healing tools and are powerful healing modalities which surpass standard therapy.

Relaxation and guided imagery also have been shown to help cancer patients deal with pain during cancer treatment. K. L. Syrjala at the Fred Hutchinson Cancer Research Center in Seattle, Washington, looked at mouth pain levels of cancer patients receiving bone marrow transplants. A total of ninety-four patients completed the study, which involved two training sessions prior to treatment and twice-a-week "booster" sessions during the first five weeks of treatment. Syrjala found that patients who received either relaxation and imagery alone reported less pain than patients who received standard allopathic care. From these results, he concluded that relaxation and imagery training reduces cancer treatment-related pain and is a useful addition to cancer care. Relaxation and guided imagery take a person "elsewhere." It takes them away from pain to a place of healing.

Guided imagery also powerfully improves the comfort of women with early-stage breast cancer undergoing radiation therapy. K. Kolcaba from the College of Nursing at the University of Akron, Ohio, studied fifty-three women with breast cancer about to begin radiation therapy. The women listened to a guided imagery audiotape once a day for the duration of the study. The study found a significant overall increase in differences in comfort levels between the treatment group and the control group, with the treatment group having higher comfort levels over time. This study showed that guided imagery is an effective intervention for enhancing the comfort of women undergoing radiation therapy for early-stage breast cancer. The intervention was especially salient in the first three weeks of therapy. Guided imagery audiotapes specifically designed for this population were found to be resource effective in terms of cost, personnel, and time.

Guided imagery also has profound effects on chemotherapy. In a similar study, L. G. Walker from the Behavioral Oncology Unit, University of Aberdeen, Medical School in Forester Hill, studied the psychological, clinical, and pathological effects of relaxation training and guided imagery during primary chemotherapy. Patients were randomized after diagnosis to a control group that used standard care or to an experimental group that used standard care plus relaxation training and imagery.

The researchers found that patients in the experimental group were more relaxed and easygoing during the study and that quality of life was better in the experimental group. The intervention also reduced emotional suppression. Finally, although the groups did not differ for clinical or pathological response to chemotherapy, imagery ratings were correlated with clinical response. Their conclusion was that relaxation and guided imagery were inexpensive and beneficial interventions and should be offered to patients wishing to improve their quality of life during primary chemotherapy. Guided imagery benefits people undergoing chemotherapy or radiation cancer treatment. Many studies such as these have demonstrated that the side effects of cancer treatment decrease with guided imagery and altered states.

Meditation has also been shown to have profound effects on healing. John Kabat-Zinn at the Stress Reduction Clinic, Center for Mindfulness in Medicine, Health Care, and Society, Department of Medicine at the University of Massachusetts Medical Center in Worcester studied the influence of a mindfulness meditation-based stress reduction intervention on skin-clearing rates in patients with moderate to severe psoriasis undergoing phototherapy and photochemotherapy. Thirty-seven patients with psoriasis about to undergo ultraviolet phototherapy or photochemotherapy were randomly assigned to one of two conditions: a mindfulness meditation-based stress reduction intervention guided by audiotaped instructions during light treatments or a control condition consisting of the light treatments alone with no taped instructions. He found that subjects in the tape groups reached the Halfway Point and the Clearing Point significantly more rapidly than those in the no-tape condition. This study showed that a brief mindfulness meditation-based stress reduction intervention delivered by audiotape during ultraviolet light therapy can increase the rate of resolution of lesions in patients with psoriasis. This sounds simple but is profound in its implications: simple meditation has been shown to affect the complex mechanisms of healing.

Finally, important studies by Diane Tusek at Cleveland Clinic in Cleveland, Ohio, demonstrate that guided imagery decreased pain and anxiety in patients having colorectal surgery. Tusek conducted a prospective, randomized trial of patients undergoing their first elective colorectal surgery at a tertiary care center. She randomly assigned patients into one of two groups. Group one received standard perioperative care, and group two listened to a guided imagery tape three days preoperatively; a music-only tape during induction, during surgery, and postoperatively in the recovery room; and a guided imagery tape during each of the first six postoperative days. Both groups had postoperative patient-controlled analgesia.

Before surgery, anxiety increased in the control group but decreased in the guided imagery group. Postoperatively, median increase in the worst pain score was 72.5 for the control group and 42.5 for the imagery group. Least pain was also significantly different, with a median increase of 30 for controls and 12.5 for the imagery group. Total opioid requirements were significantly lower in the imagery group, with a median of 185 milligrams versus 326 milligrams in the control group. Time to first bowel movement was significantly less in the imagery group (median, fifty-eight hours) than in the control group (median, ninty-two hours).

Tusek also reported the results of her recent study of patients undergoing cardiac surgery at The Cleveland Clinic Foundation. Patients who listened to the guided imagery tape had a significant decrease in pain, stress, and anxiety. These patients even left the hospital two days earlier than patients who did not listen. This groundbreaking study mandates that hospitals put guided imagery into surgery units. This kind of study will change medicine. It proves that guided imagery has significant effects on healing and is strong evidence to advise everyone to use guided imagery when they have surgery or are ill. Each hospital that did this would save millions of dollars a year by releasing patients days earlier from surgery and using less pain medication.

Perhaps most remarkably, there are studies that demonstrate that the mind affects physical reality across space and time. Dr. Robert Jahn, a former dean of engineering at Princeton University, has demonstrated that people can mentally influence the results of devices that randomly generate numbers or drop balls into slots. When volunteers try to mentally influence the patterns of these machines, the results are no longer random. Jahn has also done remote perception experiments in which a computer randomly selects a message for a volunteer to send to a receiver. The receiver then writes down the image he or she picks up, and the computer is used to analyze the image without bias. What Jahn found is that the majority of people can both send and receive thoughts, but, even more amazing, the results can be effective over a distance of 6,000 miles, and the reception can occur days before the image is even generated and sent. As an engineer, Jahn postulates material theories for how the phenomena take place, and joins an eminent group of physicists who for the last fifty years have been developing physical models to explain mind-body reality. Jahn suggests that there is a wave-mechanical resonance between sender and receiver, or electrons that tunnel through barriers, obeying the laws of quantum mechanics. Albert Einstein demonstrated in 1935 that two electrons removed from a single atom and spinning far away from each other were affected by each other's spin. This was one of the first experiments to show how objects can affect each other at a distance. Both Einstein and his fellow physicist Niels Bohr stated that matter and energy are equivalent and interchangeable, and that matter can behave as both a wave and a particle, depending on experimental conditions. Finally, the neurophysiologist Dr. Karl Pribram has postulated that mental images are like holograms, not simply like an electric circuit.

But the concept that the mind is "nonlocal," that is, that it cannot be confined to time or space, seems to be basic and still unexplainable. The physicist Erwin Schrödinger, who was instrumental in discovering quantum mechanics, tried to describe this concept: "Mind is by its very nature a singulare tantum. I should say: the over-all number of minds is just one."[2] This takes us back to the Eastern religions' concept of a great mind or power, of which everyone is a part. From this standpoint, illness could represent our ignorance of our connection with all things, and health our grasp of the one mind.

The best known study on prayer and the most challenging one to modern medicine comes from W. Harris at the Mid America Heart Institute, Saint Luke's Hospital in Kansas City, Missouri. He conducted a randomized, controlled trial of the effects of remote, intercessory prayer on outcomes in patients admitted to the coronary care unit. His objective was to determine whether remote, intercessory prayer for hospitalized, cardiac patients will reduce overall adverse events and length of stay. The research team did a randomized, controlled, double-blind, prospective, parallel-group trial. It was conducted in a private, university-associated hospital. Nine hundred ninety consecutive patients who were newly admitted to the coronary care unit were randomized to receive remote, intercessory prayer or just the usual treatment.

The first names of patients in the prayer group were given to a team of outside intercessors who prayed for them daily for four weeks. Patients were unaware that they were being prayed for, and the intercessors did not know and never met the patients. Then the researchers studied each patient's medical course from coronary care unit admission to hospital discharge. The research conclusions were that remote, intercessory prayer was associated with lower coronary care unit complication and incident scores. The result was that prayer was an effective adjunct to standard medical care. Prayer actually changed the hospital course of the patients who were prayed for. They did better and had less complications. They did not know they were being prayed for, so belief had no part in this. It was spirituality in health care at work.

Finally, we reach a subject on which little or no scientific research has been done—the spirit or soul. Traditionally this has been the realm of religion and philosophy. The brain or mind has always been difficult to comprehend, and theories about its function eventually allude to the mystical. For ages, people have believed that a part of the mind is the soul, which is connected to the great oneness. Thus the soul is both individual and universal at the same time; it is both part of a single person and part of something greater. I believe that the soul or spirit affects the mind. The soul within influences the mind, and the mind influences the body. Thus healing becomes an interplay between body, mind, and spirit. A metaphor for this interaction is that spirit frees the mind. When spirit is recognized and brought to consciousness, the mind relaxes; the mind then sends healing messages to the body. The mind is in the middle and acts as a bridge between body and spirit. The spirit must be realized or fed, or its energies cannot cross to the mind and then on to the body. Images feed the spirit, allow it to come to consciousness and flower, allow it to manifest in physical reality. The body is the mechanism by which the spirit can manifest and create. If the spirit is not recognized or fed, it wanes and can even leave the body. Traveling inward, listening to and feeding the spirit, awakens the spirit and invites it to return. It can then exert its power and force, alter the mind, and create a "new" body to do its work in the world. This model can help to explain the relationship between body, mind, and spirit. Images travel freely between body, mind, and spirit, and align or resonate with the whole. Images are the messengers from the spirit to the mind, and the mind to the spirit. They provide a two-way conversation. The spirit feeds us images to make art, and the artist produces images to feed the spirit. Awakening the soul and bringing images to consciousness free the energy of the spirit to create in the outer world. The energy that is freed helps to heal the body.

Although this discussion is theoretical, it is relevant to us for two reasons. First, it builds trust in the inner world by relating the reverie state to models that we can understand rationally and therefore believe in. Second, these models encourage us to find or create our own theories to use as a personal basis of belief.

. . .

The more we learn about healers who use guided imagery and how they work, the more we can understand and trust techniques that may seem unusual to us at first. In our efforts to heal ourselves, we eagerly take advice from people who we believe are experienced healers. In human history, the healers with the most experience in dealing with the inner world are the shaman and the Buddhist monk. Both of these figures have specialized in using the inner world for healing—the shaman for hundreds of thousands of years, the monk for thousands. The power of these healing traditions is worth our investigation. Through trial and error, both the shaman and the monk have perfected techniques that are basic to our healing work. People seem to relate easily to shamanic material, and shamanic images trigger visions and experiences of great richness. People who never heard of shamans nor had any interest in American Indian lore surprise both me and themselves by the depth of their response to shamanic material. The new popularity of shamanic rituals and material is due to the fact that this knowledge touches deep wellsprings within people and awakens symbols of our distant past. I think of this recognition as spiritual DNA, coded achetypal memories.

The term *shaman* originated in Siberia and Central Asia. It refers to a priest/healer/magician who was a master of the reverie state. In my view of the history of imagery, humans have gone through several ages of interacting with the inner world. In the first age, all people were able to enter the reverie state and see and talk to spirits. Everyone saw the world as alive, as populated with spirits, and as a single whole of which they were a part. Thus to them, all the world was sacred space. But they could enter even more deeply into the sacred space or the inner world by specific techniques that usually involved dancing, drumming, or taking herbs that contained mind-altering substances. During these inner journeys, people would see the spirits more clearly and interact with them more directly.

At the dawn of history people probably didn't even need these aids to see spirits. But as time went on, people became increasingly separated from the inner world. Because they were concentrating more on the outer or material world, they needed more help to make contact with the spirits. Finally, most people lost their ability to see the spirits, although there always remained a small group who were good at it. These people, through dreams, visions, and even illness, would spontaneously see spirits, and often would then devote their life to perfecting this ability. Thus the role of shaman, or specialist in the inner world, arose. Because shamans frequently began by healing themselves of an illness, which they saw as a spiritual disharmony, healing became the main practical use of shamanic skill.

In fact, throughout almost all of human history and in almost all cultures, the cause of physical illness was believed to be basically spiritual. It was attributed to losing one's spirit or soul, having one's spirit tampered with by another person, or being out of harmony with the sacred, or inner, world. It is only Western industrial culture that has believed that, in general, illness is physically caused. It is interesting to note that this view is undergoing change in light of the growth of the new mind-body medicine. Whether this history of humankind and the inner world is factual or mythological is questionable. Certainly the myth of the fall from paradise that is found in many cultures portrays a world in which people lost the ability to contact the spirits directly. For us, this history has great relevance because people are once again attempting to heal themselves through inner journeys. Thus, in a sense, we are relearning what human beings knew at the dawn of history.

The shaman healed by going into a trance or reverie state, traveling to sacred regions, and interacting with the spirits to make the patient's soul whole. The shaman either brought the lost soul back or talked the evil spirits into letting go of the person's soul. So, in a real sense, the shaman was an expert on the inner world and the human soul. In our times, healers who work with guided imagery have resisted taking on these tasks. It has been more common for healers to teach people to embark on inner journeys themselves and thus share in the role of the shaman. When a shaman was involved in a healing, he or she would often describe the inner journey in great detail, so that the patient and everyone participating could share in the vision to some extent. But the basic belief of the people was probably that the shaman, not the patient, performed the healing. This part of the inner world is confusing to most people schooled in scientific reality.

For ages it has been believed that images held in one person's mind could actually be instrumental in healing another person. Thus, when a shaman "saw" a person's soul and brought it back, he or she was able to facilitate some sort of change in that person's physiology. The current term for this phenomenon is *transpersonal imagery*. I will talk more about this concept in Chapter 7. Transpersonal imagery lies at the heart of healing circles, prayer circles, and even something as common as sitting at a sick person's bedside and envisioning him or her getting better. As difficult as it may be to explain scientifically, transpersonal imagery is understandable within the laws of the inner world. There boundaries between people are not fixed, and thoughts create reality. The concept of the shaman has great relevance for us in terms of awakening our healing spirit. The shaman has always been a symbol of a channel of power from the inner world. Each of us has a part of our mind that can function as our own shaman. It is a part of our mind that is the same as the mind of the shaman throughout all ages.

When the shaman heals, he or she goes into a reverie state and travels into the inner world. The shaman views the inner world as having its own landmarks and features, which are referred to as *sacred geography*. One cannot prove whether it is literal rather than symbolic, but it is useful. The inner world is viewed by shamans from some cultures as having three levels, or *cosmic zones:* the *sky,* the *earth,* and the *lower world.* These levels are connected by a central axis. The central axis passes through an opening or hole and provides a means for moving from one level to another. The hole, which is in the center, is the site of a breakthrough in plane. The shaman believes that the gods and spirits come to earth from above or below by passing through the hole. Celestial figures or gods are believed to be in the sky, while the spirits of the dead and animal spirits are found in the lower world. The axis is often represented in myth as a tree, a bridge, a staircase, a sacred mountain, or the central pole of a dwelling. The top of the axis is often represented as the Pole Star. Commonly, the mountain has seven (or nine) levels, the tree that number of branches. The shaman travels in these unknown regions with the aid of guardian spirits. Shamans believe that many animals and objects and natural phenomena have spirits that can confer help and power. These spirits are believed to be essential for the shaman's journey. Without their guidance, the shaman would become lost in the inner world.

Often shamans discovered their powers as a result of being ill, but they always had a dream or vision. In the vision, they would be taken to the sky or the lower world, and initiated. A primary part of the initiation involved the shaman's own death and dismemberment. The shaman's body would be stripped down to bone and the skeleton thrown to the winds. Then helpers or teachers would build a new body. Upon returning to the earth, the shaman would be healed and have the power to heal. In a symbolic sense, we can say that as a result of this journey, shamans become empowered. They receive power from the earth through animal helpers, and power from the sky through guardian helpers or tutelary spirits, and thus are made whole and can find their path. In a real sense, illness played a transformative role in the shaman's lives. The loss of soul that made the shamans ill made them feel weak and powerless. The return of their soul gives the shamans back power and energy. Through this journey, the shamans gain access to deep parts of the mind that had the memories of animal powers. By merging and becoming one with these animals, the shamans can enter the part of their inner world that has healing energy.

The Buddhist monk took imagery and inner journeys even further. Monks visualized pantheons of celestial figures in tremendous detail. In order to do this, the monks would go into a reverie state, picture a deity in its celestial realm, and then imagine that the picture moved to various parts of their body and merged with it. They would imagine the image becoming as large as possible, as large as the universe, and then as small as a sesame seed. They would imagine the deity changing color and becoming vacuous or empty, and they would consciously hold the image of the deity in their mind for long periods of time. The primary goal of these practices was not healing but spiritual growth or enlightenment. Buddhist monks believe that by repeating exercises that have been perfected over thousands of years, they could reach enlightenment and gain true knowledge of the universe. Along the way, the exercises would exert powerful effects on the body's physiology and heal illness. These are the most elaborately worked out imagery techniques that we have at our disposal. Unlike the techniques of the shaman, they involve conscious control of the inner world. Whereas the shaman waits for things to happen on an inner journey, the monk deliberately creates forms and manipulates them.

In contemporary imagery for healing, we utilize the techniques of both the shaman and the monk. We use the shaman's experiences to help us journey into the inner world and there find power animals, celestial figures, and inner guides. This aspect of contemporary healing gives us access to our own healing power through the symbols that it frees inside us. We use the monk's experiences to help us hold healing images in order to change our body's physiology. Instead of concentrating on celestial figures, most physicians and psychologists using imagery have their patients picture their illness and their healing mechanisms and focus on an image of those healing mechanisms, eliminating the illness and repairing the body. Most commonly, people picture anatomical representations and physiological processes. In that sense, these are material visualizations. With time, the images usually become more metaphorical and symbolic. Because they come from a person's own inner center, they develop greater energy. As the images increase in power, they have more direct effects on body physiology and promote greater healing.

The Discussion

Now we will work on building skills; we will learn about and practice the three basic techniques of the reverie state: relaxation, meditation, and guided imagery. These skills are both enjoyable and powerful; they can help us deal with worry and stress, make our bodies stronger, and heal illness. When people do these exercises for the first time, they are amazed by the new experiences they have. A woman with high blood pressure who had never consciously worked in the reverie state said that after her first relaxation exercise, her body felt "new." She felt that a great tension had released itself and that she had opened up. She said that for the first time she felt at home in her body, and understood for the first time that she didn't have to keep her muscles clenched. Profound feelings of relaxation give people an instant respite from the problems of their life. The physical pleasure derived from relaxation techniques is extraordinary. Meditation produces a calmness and feeling of power that is difficult to achieve any other way. For many people, guided imagery actually opens up a new world within. Initially, people have the most trouble with guided imagery because they believe it is difficult. However, you will see that imagery is a simple type of experience that you actually have all the time when you daydream.

The goal of the exercises in this chapter is to teach you how to enter and work in the reverie state. Relaxation is necessary for most inner journeys. By itself, deep relaxation changes our focus from outer to inner and produces an altered state of consciousness. The relaxed state also quiets the sympathetic nervous system and changes our physiology. It reduces our perception of pain and enhances our feelings of well-being. Relaxation involves more complex and profound changes than simply eliminating muscle tension. It acts as a doorway into the reverie state and relieves worries and fears, detaching us from daily concerns. In general, relaxation is the easiest way for Westerners to get into the healing state.

Whereas relaxation has predominated as the basic reverie tool in the West, meditation has long been fundamental to all inner work in the East. Recently Westerners have also discovered that meditation is a powerful tool for healing. Meditation clears and relaxes the mind. It acts directly on our thinking processes, and its power is limitless. Meditation helps us gain control over our thoughts so that we are not prey to constant anxieties, fears, and worries. For people with an illness that they think about

continuously, this is a real gift. At a deeper level, beyond controlling our thoughts, meditation teaches us to focus our mind on
whatever we choose. In the case of healing, meditation allows us
to focus on thoughts or images that automatically produce healing. Focusing on these images relieves pain and increases energy.
At the deepest levels, meditation allows us to glimpse realms that
reveal our connections with everything in the universe, including
the creative force behind nature. Experiencing such feelings is the
most profound healing. This state of union is an ideal state; it is
the goal of most people on a spiritual journey. In a sense, the healing that accompanies this state is a secondary effect of enlightenment, rather than the primary goal. In terms of this book, healing
may be a person's primary goal, at least initially, but the path is the
same.

Finally, in guided imagery we take the relaxed or meditative
state and use it to concentrate on images in our inner world. In
guided imagery, we use all five inner senses, we live and feel the
experience. The inner experience is real, but it is completely different from an outer world experience. It feels like a daydream as
opposed to a perception. The inner world is as rich and full as the
outer, but softer and more subtle. The key to the guided imagery
experience is to realize that when you are doing or seeing something in your mind, and are using your senses in an internal way,
you are imaging.

The Exercises

Exercise 2—Basic Relaxation.

Find a comfortable space where you will not be disturbed. Sit
or lie down with your legs uncrossed, your arms at your sides
or resting on your abdomen. Loosen any tight or constricting
clothing. Close your eyes. Begin by inhaling slowly and deeply
through your nostrils. Let the breath out through the nose
slowly and completely. Continue breathing in this manner,
allowing your abdomen to rise as you inhale and fall as you

exhale. As you breathe allow yourself to relax. Let your consciousness float behind your nostrils and feel the air going in and out of your nose. Now shift your consciousness to your feet and allow them to relax. Concentrate on feelings of tingling, buzzing, pulsing, warmth or coolness, heaviness or lightness. Now let your ankles relax. Allow the feelings of relaxation to spread up the back of your legs. Now allow your calves to relax. Continue to breathe in and out slowly, and let the feelings of relaxation deepen. Allow your knees to relax, and the muscles of your thighs. While you're relaxing, let your mind float free, momentarily alighting on the feeling of air moving through your nostrils, then concentrating on the particular part of your body you are relaxing. Take a moment and release any worries or anxieties you may have. Release them—you don't need them—and let them drift away. If you wish, you may watch them float off as you exhale. You can name the particular worry and see it slip away as a bubble, a dark area, or a bird. All you're doing here is allowing your body to relax; it knows how to do this by itself.

Now allow your pelvic area to relax. Feel the relaxation in your genitals, anus, and buttocks. Release the tension that everyone carries in their pelvis. Now let your abdomen relax. Allow it to relax as it rises and falls; allow your breathing to take place by itself. Allow the muscles of your chest to relax. Let your breath go in and out smoothly; allow your breathing to take place by itself. Let your heartbeat be smooth and regular. Let your mind float over your entire body. Concentrate on feelings of buzzing, vibrating, tingling, lightness, or heaviness. You may notice that your body feels as if it were getting larger or that space seems to be expanding. You may also notice that the inside of your body seems hollow and large and that your entire consciousness seems quiet and deep.

Allow the feelings of relaxation that you are experiencing to spread into your shoulders. Let your shoulders relax; let them drop. Now let your upper arms relax, and let the feeling spread to your lower arms and hands. Feel the sensations of tingling and numbness spread through your hands, and let your mind wander back over your body, down to your feet, deepening the relaxation throughout your whole body. Now let your neck relax. Let the big muscles that support your head loosen and lengthen. Now let the feelings of relaxation spread up to your head. Relax your scalp, let your jaw drop, let the muscles around your eyes relax, and let your forehead relax.

Now concentrate on a place on the top of your head. You may feel tingling or buzzing there. As you take a breath, allow energy to flow into your body through that area, and allow your body to expand. Imagine that millions of moving particles of light come into your body through the top of your head, go down along your spine, and move out to envelop your whole body. Enjoy these feelings of relaxation. It almost seems as if your body disappears and your consciousness is floating outside your body, in front of your eyes. Now direct your attention to any areas of your body that feel tense or that bother you. Let them relax; let them drop. Allow the energy coming in through your head to flow to those areas, move around them, and caress them. Allow the energy to go through them and fill them with light. Remain in this wonderfully relaxed state as long as you wish.

When you wish to return to your everyday state, gently move your feet and count slowly from one to three. Press your feet down toward the floor and feel the sensations of your muscles tensing. You will return to your everyday state relaxed, comfortable, and full of energy. Your body will feel as if it is in a comfortable, healing space. Each time you do this exercise you will relax more deeply and more easily. The feelings of relaxation will deepen, and the whole exercise will become more and more pleasurable.

What was this exercise like? How did you feel? Generally people enjoy deep relaxation; however, some people may feel as if nothing happened, or they may have felt bored. Some people feel that they simply cannot relax and are constantly occupied with thoughts about their everyday life. First, biofeedback studies have shown that everyone can relax. Even if you are not aware of sensations of relaxation, doctors can see and measure relaxation taking place in your muscles. Even if you didn't feel that anything was happening, trust that you are relaxing and try to tune in to the subtle feelings that signal relaxation. If boredom was a problem during this exercise, do not be concerned because upcoming exercises will be taken up with guided imagery and will be more active. Most people who do this exercise are amazed by how pleasurable it is. Relaxation by itself releases worries. Many people report wanting to stay in the relaxation space and not come back to their everyday world. Sometimes people spontaneously start to image when they relax. Occasionally people will fall asleep during the relaxation exercise, especially if they are very tired or the room is darkened. This is not a problem. Repeat the exercise when you are less tired. Finally, some people, when they are deeply relaxed, will experience the sensations of floating and may even feel as if their consciousness is outside of their physical body. These are common experiences, which become more profound as people relax more and more deeply.

Exercise 3—Beginning Meditation.

Find a comfortable space where you will not be disturbed. Sit on a chair or cushion with your ankles crossed, your back straight, and your arms resting on your abdomen. Loosen any tight or constricting clothing. Close your eyes. Begin by inhaling slowly and deeply through your nostrils. Let the breath out through your nose slowly and completely. Continue breathing in this manner, allowing your abdomen to rise as you inhale and fall as you exhale. As you breathe allow yourself to relax. Now simply concentrate on the sensation of air moving in and out at the tips of your nostrils. Concentrate only on the sensations at the end of your nostrils. If you wish, you can say "in" or "one" as you're breathing in, and "out" or "two" as you're exhaling. You can concentrate on the sensations of air moving in your nose, windpipe, or chest. Or you can concentrate on your abdomen rising and falling and say to yourself "rising" and "falling" as you breathe in and out.

The goal of this exercise is simply to concentrate on the sensations or verbal signals. If other thoughts come to mind, simply return your attention to the breathing when you notice your attention has wandered. Everyone's mind wanders. This is natural. With practice, your mind will wander less. If you wish, you can note the type of thought that interrupts your concentration and say to yourself "sound," "worry," "judgment," "ideas," "images." Naming the thought takes the emotion from it and allows you to go rapidly back to your counting or breathing. If you wish, you can stop the extraneous thought as soon as you notice it, or you can allow yourself to complete the idea or sentence. As you watch your breathing, you'll notice that you become calmer and more peaceful, that your inner space expands, and that you become alert but quiet, watchful yet detached.

The next part of this exercise involves sending love to all beings and the universe. You'll start with yourself and work outward. First, meditate on the positive aspects of yourself. Repeat thoughts mentally, pause, and watch your breath. Start by giving yourself the message "I love myself." Repeat this phrase several times. If you wish, you can picture yourself as you do this. Next list your strong points, one at a time; repeat each several times. "I love my courage, intelligence, generosity, ability to help, warmth, loving nature, perseverance, parenting skills, work abilities"—whatever qualities you have that make you feel good and make your life and others' lives better. You can do this as long as you wish; there is no time limit. The more things you can think of the better. Next, say to yourself, "I love my body." Think of all the enjoyable, positive things about your body and what you do well in a physical sense. For example: "I love my strength, coordination, agility, ability to run, the good feelings I get when I lie in the sun, my smile, the way I walk, the way my hair looks, the size and shape of my hands." As you meditate on these aspects of yourself, you can concentrate on the images that they evoke. End by sending love to your body and mind.

Now, repeat the same process with other people: Start

with the person closest to you and work outward to those you know less well. Most people start with their partner or a close friend, go on to their children, and then move to their parents and other relatives. In each case, think about the positive characteristics, mental and physical, of those people. End with each person by sending love out to that individual and letting the energy envelop him or her.

Next, concentrate on the positive aspects of the place where you live and the people who live near you. Again, end by sending out waves of love to the people and the place. Work outward from your neighborhood to your city, your county, your state, your country, your continent, the earth, and the universe. Meditate on whatever positive image is evoked by these words. Try to see an overall picture, almost like an aerial photograph. And don't move on to the next category until you surround the present one with love.

Now imagine that many people are doing the same meditation as you at the same time, and picture the positive energy that it produces. Feel your interconnectedness with these other people. Visualize in your own mind how your energy and love merge with that of all the other people. Now imagine that you are interconnected with all the objects and all the beings in the universe. Imagine that a thread comes from your heart and joins with a similar thread from all the other creatures to make a ball of light. Finally, imagine that your love and energy make this light become brighter and brighter.

People are continually amazed by how simple yet how difficult meditation is. In fact, five minutes of meditation is a workout. For most people it requires a high level of concentration. Everyone loses track of their breathing at some point, no matter how hard they try. When you lose track, you realize that you are not in control of your thoughts. Most of us believe our will is in control of our thoughts and are extremely surprised to discover that our thoughts seem to come by themselves. After practicing meditation, we can begin to see our thoughts as soon as they arise, and we are able to return to our breathing that much more quickly. Such meditation practice enables us to gain greater control over our imagery. Some people find breath meditation problematic. They lose track immediately or get bored or sleepy. This is normal for some people and need not be a problem. It is important to realize that people's skills improve with practice, and if they persevere, the meditation will become easier. The benefits of meditation occur by themselves. Even if it seems difficult, it is not necessary to do anything other than the exercise. I have found meditation techniques so useful that I teach them to anyone who has trouble holding images because of intrusive thoughts. It is especially valuable when people are ill and find it hard to get their mind off their worries.

The meditation that we just did is extremely calming and reassuring. In effect, it allows you to be your own support system. It also makes you feel secure. The love and connectedness it brings forth are basic and fulfilling; thus the meditation increases a person's power and strength. It is especially useful when someone is anxious, afraid, or worried, because it allows the person to eliminate negative energy without having to confront the cause of it. This kind of loving state is intimately connected with the healing state.

Many people merge meditation with prayer and pray to whatever powers they believe in. A deep altered state of consciousness results from the combination of prayer and meditation. Often people's prayers draw them out of themselves, connecting them to something greater than themselves. This experience relaxes boundaries and increases their sense of interconnectedness.

Most people report that this exercise increases their feelings of love, warmth, and connectedness. At the same time it reduces fear and worry. The meditation also increases self-confidence and a sense of personal power. It is such a basic and useful exercise that it can be used to counter many of the problems that can occur during guided imagery work, including distraction, fear, loss of control, and loss of self-confidence. A physician I worked with worried continuously about his work. He often felt that he was ineffective and was not valuable to his patients. He felt that he could never do enough or do his work perfectly. Meditation proved to be a great help to him. During his daily meditation he would list as many strong points about himself as he could think of and would feel his sense of power increase. This sense of greater strength would last for most of the day. When he would meditate on his family and friends, he would feel increasing well-being and a sense of energy. After the exercise he would feel more awake and ready to start his day with a sense of connectedness and peace. After meditating he would understand that he was who he was and that his positivity and healing manner helped his patients greatly.

Exercise 4—Beginning Guided Imagery.

Find a comfortable space where you will not be disturbed. Sit or lie down with your legs uncrossed, your arms at your sides or resting on your abdomen. Loosen any tight or constricting clothing. Close your eyes. Begin by inhaling slowly and deeply through your nostrils. Let the breath out through the nose slowly and completely. Continue breathing in this manner, allowing your abdomen to rise as you inhale and fall as you exhale. As you breathe allow yourself to relax. Let yourself relax completely. Release any worries or tensions that you have; let them float off. Let the feeling of relaxation spread throughout your body. (If you feel it is necessary, repeat Exercise 2, Basic Relaxation.)

Now imagine that you are in a room you are comfortable in. It may be a room in the place where you live, work, or grew up. Imagine that you are in the middle of the room on a bright sunny day. Give yourself a moment to get used to your surroundings. Glance around the room. Notice the doors, the windows, the floor and ceiling, and any furniture in the room. Let your eyes take in the objects in the room; scan them. Now mentally zoom in on any piece of furniture and concentrate on the details. Look at what it is made out of, its style and carving. Look at the surface; now touch it and feel its texture. Is it rough or smooth, warm or cold? Now zoom in on other objects in your room. See what the windowsills and curtains are made of. Look closely at the other furniture. Let your eyes travel and take in details. Notice scratches or chips in paint, light reflections, and shiny areas. Touch the windowsill or furniture. Feel the texture of the material from which they are made. Smell the air in the room. Does it have a particular odor of wood, perfume, or flowers? Listen for any sounds in the room. Is there a clock ticking, are there noises coming from the rest of the house or from outside? Get as vivid a picture of the room as you can.

Now in your mind's eye, imagine making changes in the room. Because this is in your imagination, you can make any changes you wish. First, mentally rearrange the furniture. Try the furniture in a number of different locations. If you wish, remove some of the furniture entirely or add new pieces. Now imagine that the walls of the room change color. Choose any colors or wallpaper that you wish. Also, imagine that the floor is different. Pick any kind of rug, hardwood floor, or tile. Each time you make a change, you can let it go or you can keep it. Now imagine that the windows or doors change shape or position. You might make the windows larger or move them to a different place on the wall; you might make them out of a different material or architectural style. Finally, you might change the shape or size of the room. You could expand the room, make it round, or change the ceiling. Make changes in your room for as long as you wish.

Now let your room return to its original state. Pause a moment and look around. Get comfortable. Now imagine that someone you love or respect, a family member, close friend, healer, or teacher is coming to visit you in your room. You can invite anyone you wish, or even let the person who comes be a surprise to you. Look up when that person knocks at the door, and watch as he or she enters the room. Notice what the person is wearing and how he or she walks. Greet the person and listen for a reply. Begin a conversation. In your imagination, tell the person that you're happy to see him or her, and talk as if the person really was in the room with you.

When you finish speaking, pause and hear what the person says in return. It will seem to you like the other side of an inner conversation with yourself. You can talk about a shared interest or ask any questions you wish. You may want to tell the person something that you haven't been able to share before. Continue the conversation as long as you wish. Say good-bye and watch as the person leaves your room.

Now imagine that your room undergoes a radical change and becomes a place to begin a journey. Let all the furniture disappear. Let the ceiling and the roof lift off, exposing the sky. Let the walls fold out. You are now on a platform with the sky above you. Imagine that you start to float upward from the platform, rising at a faster and faster speed until you are soaring. The space around you is now turning dark, and stars begin to appear. Continue rising into the dark, starry sky. In front of you, in the distance, you will see an area of white light. The area is bright but so far away that it appears to be only several feet in diameter. Allow yourself to drift toward the light. Notice the stars moving past you as you drift. As you move toward it the area of white light becomes larger and larger. Finally it begins to fill your whole field. Allow yourself to drift into the center of the light. Feel the light around you. Imagine the light is made up of millions of dots of moving energy. Imagine that the dots of energy can move through your body easily, as if it were not solid. Now feel the light and energy inside you as well as around you. Feel yourself become one with the light and its energy. If any areas of your body attract your attention, allow the light and energy to increase there. Rest in the healing peace of the light as long as you wish.

When you wish to return to your everyday state, gently move your feet, press them to the floor, and count slowly from one to three. You will return to your everyday state relaxed, comfortable, and full of energy. Your body will feel as if it is in a comfortable, healing space. Each time you do this exercise you will relax more deeply and more easily. The feelings of relaxation will deepen, and the whole exercise will become more and more pleasurable.

. . .

This exercise is somewhat similar to the guided imagery exercise we used in Chapter 1. The imagery is similar, but here we have started to purposefully build skills. Some of you may have realized by this point that guided imagery is something you do all the time. Other people may be frustrated and feel that they are unable to image. One woman I worked with was a powerful and intuitive person who had strong body feelings about people and things going on around her. She had a lifelong interest in psychology and the inner world. She believed that she could get in touch with inner sounds, but she never was able to see images. After this exercise she was frustrated and discouraged. She came up to me and told me she could not image, and asked me for advice. I had her picture the letter "A" and imagine drawing around the letter and tracing its outlines. I told her to see the letter in her mind's eye as she was doing this. I asked her if she could sense the letter or see it. She said, "Of course, but is that all imagery is?" She had expected her imagery to be as real as a movie or an outer scene. Imagery is just a mental picture. The more you do it, the more vivid and real it becomes. But in the beginning, it is like tracing the letter "A"—no more or less than that. This simple experience enabled the woman to realize that she could image constantly, that images were all around her in her inner world. She said that I had given her a magic apple. From that point on, she had vivid imagery experiences that became more and more intense and meaningful.

Another common complaint of people who are starting to work with images is that they are distracted by certain instructions in the exercise that cause them to get off track. One woman that I worked with could not imagine a room in her house because she had just separated from her husband and the thought of her home was upsetting. One man had just moved and couldn't decide which house he should image. My advice during guided imagery exercises is to allow your own imagery to arise. If a phrase or direction disturbs you, simply ignore it and make up your own. Both of the people who had trouble picturing a room in their house had no trouble picturing another room elsewhere. They got stuck when I mentioned their house, and could go no further. The important thing is to get back on the exercise when you've fallen off. Grab on to anything you can and keep going.

One psychologist I worked with got stuck in the "room where you grew up" phrase. He had had an unhappy childhood, and that phrase brought up memories of his discomfort. While I did the rest of the exercise, he could not concentrate and became increasingly uncomfortable. Finally he found a part that appealed to him: when I talked about "white light," he felt much better. During any imagery exercise, if you start to feel uncomfortable and think about other thoughts, simply stop. Concentrate on your breathing, let the negative thoughts out, and try to focus on something else in the exercise. If you still cannot do the exercise, imagine a pleasant scene, let yourself relax, and don't chastise yourself. You don't have to complete every part of any of the exercises.

For some people visual and sound images are not very strong but body feelings are intense. Throughout this book there will be many different types of exercises. Some will be natural for you and will provoke intense feelings. Some may be difficult and frustrating. Concentrate on the exercises that are natural and easy for you; the others will come. Congratulate yourself for what you've started to do. Each time you work on guided imagery exercises you will get better.

3

THE JOURNEY: ATTITUDES AND PERSONAL MYTHS

In my work with patients and workshop participants, I see great beauty in everyone. Each person has a different worldview, but all of us share a common thread: a need to change, create, grow, and heal. If the reverie state is the vehicle for going inward, it is our attitude and view of the world that help to determine the path that we travel. I view healing as a journey—a journey that takes us from darkness into light. Now that we have learned basic imagery skills, we are ready to begin to use them. The first step is to consider our attitude or worldview. This large image makes up our orientation, our outlook, and our myth.

Researchers are now discovering that attitudes are key to health. Attitude helps determine how we perceive discomfort and how we heal. Our attitude has an impact on the side effects of medication and is fundamental to anxiety and depression. A nurse I worked with had just left her job and felt depressed and lost. Her job had been stressful, and she felt she was a failure. One day during an imagery exercise she saw herself from afar. She saw her negativity and depression and realized that she could choose her mental state. When she finished the exercise, she realized that she could choose to feel powerless and concentrate on those feelings, or she could choose a more positive viewpoint. She felt that this exercise changed her life. Afterward she was able to act consciously to see herself in control. She purposely began to choose activities and pursuits that she enjoyed and made her happy. She decided to get a degree in art therapy and work with children, and each day became more enjoyable.

Whether or not we have an illness, we are all traveling on a path toward an unseen goal. That goal is unique for each person. And no one knows just where it comes from. Perhaps we are born with it, perhaps it is the result of experiences that happen to us, perhaps it is given to us by a greater force. Perhaps it comes from our soul or inner center. Each of us has a part to play in life; each of us has a gift, something to contribute. Our collective goal or collective purpose is unknown to most of us and is tied to the movement of the whole universe. The universe itself is creative and is growing. The center of each of us is connected to the creative center of the universe. The flow of creativity from each one of us is part of the growth of the huge entity that is the universe. Glimpsing our creative place in the universe helps us form positive attitudes and gives us a reason for being.

This chapter is about attitude and myth. By attitude, I mean underlying philosophies or worldviews. By myth, I mean the story of the basics of our philosophy in symbol form. This book is, in a real sense, my own attitude, worldview, or myth. My attitude here is assembled from science, religion, philosophy, and my experience with people with illnesses. It has power in that it helps me heal and gives me stability when I'm afraid. It is useful to me. The sources of our myths are our ancestors—our teachers. The source is our culture. We have access now, for the first time in history, to the whole culture of humankind—not just the story of our people in a limited sense, but the story of our people in the broadest sense. Each of us must make our myth visible.

A person's philosophy is one of the basic determinants of the path he or she takes. Our philosophy affects all the choices we make. Almost more important than that, our philosophy affects how we view events. Joseph Campbell, who devoted his life to studying myth and religion, evolved a philosophy of joy and inner growth expressed in his maxim "Follow your bliss." Not only does that attitude help people make choices, but I believe that it is intimately involved in keeping people healthy. The aphorism "Follow your bliss" is a basic healing tool. Using it as a guide leads people to make one choice after another based on how they feel. By "bliss," I do not mean instant pleasure; rather, as I use the term, "bliss" refers to the creative energy that is released when we listen to the voice of our inner center, the part of ourselves that is beyond ego and is in harmony with the world around us. To follow your bliss means to follow the voice of your inner center.

The inner center, spirit, or soul is our individual part of the force of life. It is the doorway to something greater than ourselves. It is still individual in that it reflects our individual path, whether it be as healer, artist, community worker, or other role, but it is universal in that it serves the needs of the universal organism at the same time. The inner Self is a concept that has been dealt with by philosophers throughout the ages. The Greeks called it *daimon,* the Egyptians called it *ba-sol,* and the Romans called it *genius.* Nonliterate societies often referred to it as a protective spirit. Frequently it was seen as an animal spirit. In these societies, people talked to their inner spirit like an inner voice. The Naskapi Indians of northern Canada believe that the inner center is an inner companion called the Great Man. The Great Man guided the Naskapi with instructions and images. The Naskapi believe that generosity and love attract the Great Man and that lies and dishonesty drive the Great Man away. Carl Jung had a similar concept he called the Self. He believed that the Self was an organizing center that regulated and directed our lives, which was "the inventor, organizer, and source of dream images."[1] Jung believed that the Self was at the same time both the nucleus of the psyche and the whole psyche, and that the ego was a tiny reflection on the surface of the Self.

In this book I will refer to the Self as the *inner center;* I believe it is homeostatic and health-producing. The inner center balances the different parts of the body with each other, and balances the body with the world around it. But it can only do so if people are attuned to its voice. The ego is powerful enough that it often blocks out the voice of the inner center. Unlike the inner center, the ego can do things that are harmful to a person. The ego, like a young child, often sees only its own point of view.

Reverie is the means by which we will glimpse our inner center. Many of our attitudes and philosophies derive from the inner center. Our attitudes are like giant images. They color and control all aspects of our life. They are the dominant thoughts and images that govern all our reactions. I refer to these basic attitudes as *mega-images*. What medicine is discovering is that, in general, positive attitudes help to create health and heal, whereas negative attitudes make illness more likely and healing more difficult. I believe that positive attitudes flow from the inner center, and negative attitudes from the ego's conditioning by society. Positive and negative attitudes provide us with another paradox to be resolved. They are a pair of opposites, both of which help us work toward growth. Just as pain and suffering are teachers for us, so is bliss. The difference is that holding and concentrating on negative emotions can result in illness, while bliss can heal.

I help people to heal themselves by encouraging them to pay attention to their inner messages. Negative messages alert us to make changes and can keep us on our path, but the ultimate goal is reached through positive messages. At every moment of our lives, we can choose to hold positive attitudes, we can concentrate on love rather than fear, on those things that bring us joy and delight rather than worry, on happiness rather than depression. This chapter is about consciously choosing and acting upon positive attitudes. The most basic positive attitude is our will to live. This attitude comes naturally from our inner center, but it can be suppressed by the ego's sadnesses and the problems of life. Focusing only on ourselves as separate, it is easy for us to become confused and lose sight of our inner center. Dispelling this confusion and sadness is crucial to health. Dr. Larry LeShan, a psychotherapist who has worked with many cancer patients, says that the body mobilizes its self-healing and self-recuperative powers when a person with cancer begins to search for his or her "own unique song." When we find our inner voice, our will to live is freed, and this influences all our actions.

Our philosophy of life, our worldview, plays a tremendous role in whether or not we get ill and in how we deal with illness. The mind has powerful effects on the body's physiological processes. In the last chapter I described how pleasurable images result in the healing physiology of the relaxation response, whereas fearful images cause the fight-or-flight response by creating sympathetic arousal. An image of a pleasurable scene or an image of a fearful scene is simple and straightforward. In reality, the images and thoughts that we process are often much more complicated. In this chapter I will explain how the complex images that constitute our attitude affect our health. Knowledge is the key to control; information is useful in that it broadens your understanding of the spirit/mind/body connection. Studies about attitude reinforce your intuitive feelings and provide motivation to make changes in attitude and lifestyle. The studies that I'll talk about make up the current scientific myth about mind/body healing.

The first studies that made doctors aware of the link between attitude and health had to do with stress. At first, stress was looked upon as a simple concept that referred to events that caused people to become anxious or upset. As stated earlier, research not only links stress with disease, but has actually been able to pinpoint the physiological mechanisms by which the stress response takes place. One classic study showed that during final exams, students had lowered immune function, including diminished natural killer cell and helper T cell activity. In animal studies, stressful events such as overcrowding, excessive noise, exposure to a predator, and shock were shown to lower the functioning of the immune system and make it more likely that the animal would develop an infection or cancer. The phrase "more likely" is the key here. Illness is caused by a combination of factors, including our genetics, our environment, and our attitude. Each of these aspects plays a different role, and each person has different thresholds for different diseases at different times. Even if attitude did not play a major role in becoming ill in certain circumstances, it can play an important role in healing.

The more researchers study stress and illness, the more complex the relationship appears to be. Recent definitions of stress explain the concept in terms of a person's perception of a particular event. That is, what is stressful to one person may not be stressful to another. For example, the psychologist David Ornstein and the physician David Sobel say that "the way we perceive and appraise the event, the availability and use of resources to cope with the challenge, have more to do with the outcome than the raw event itself. Stress, and its negative impact on health, derive from a mismatch between perceived environmental demands and perceived resources to adapt."[2] The stress-researcher Milton Kaplan goes even further in terms of considering a person's whole life. He states that stress is "the inability of the individual to obtain meaningful information that his actions are leading to desired consequences."[3] In other words, stress results from the sense that your actions won't achieve your goals. It is clear that these new definitions of stress involve a person's attitudes as much or more than they involve an external event. Stress begins to be viewed as an inner phenomenon rather than an outer event.

Stress studies show that the physiological changes brought about by stress are linked to people's perception of their control over a situation. When people believe that their actions will have an effect on a situation, they do not feel as helpless as people who believe their actions are useless. The effects of helplessness on health have been shown in several animal studies. In one study, two groups of mice were subjected to the same mild electric shock. Of the two groups, one was able to stop the shocks by pressing a lever in the cage, whereas the other group had no means of controlling the shocks. Researchers found that tumors introduced onto the skin of the mice grew much more rapidly and were less likely to be rejected by the mice who were unable to control the shocks, even though the number of shocks received by the two groups was the same. Other studies have shown that rats have decreased immune function when they receive uncontrollable shock, yet have normal immune function when they receive shock they can control. Researchers refer to the attitude induced by uncontrollable stress as *learned helplessness*. These studies have important implications for people who feel helpless or hopeless in facing an illness. The message these studies convey is that it is useful to work toward increasing our power and control. We do this, in part, by changing our attitude.

The next piece in the puzzle that links health and attitudes involves the remarkable role that support plays in countering stress and producing health. When people receive help their perception of stressful events somehow changes and they are less likely to become ill and more likely to heal. Katherine Nuckolls's classic study of pregnant women and complications of pregnancy found that among two groups of pregnant women, both of whom experienced high stress, the group with greater intimacy and support had lower rates of complications. Since the Nuckolls study, a number of other studies have demonstrated that support reduces mortality and job absenteeism and lowers the incidence of heart disease and cancer. The study by Spiegel discussed in the previous chapter even indicated that support increased longevity for patients with breast cancer. Thus contact with sympathetic people alters our body's response to disease.

Even more recently, researchers have found that people deal with stress in various ways. We all know people who are generally worriers and others who are basically at peace with themselves. Stress researchers say those people who appear to deal with stress more effectively have good *coping* skills. Studies have begun to examine what enables people to cope with stress. The first studies were done by the behavioral psychologist Richard Lazarus, who theorized that when people experience a life event, they appraise the situation to see if they need to act on it, and if they do, they then assess whether or not they have the resources to deal with it. Lazarus believes that people perceive events as either a challenge or a threat. If they see a situation as threatening, they will feel stress. The Stanford University psychologist Albert Bandura conducted a study whose results supported Lazarus's thesis. Bandura took a group of women who were afraid of spiders and gave them tasks that involved handling spiders. Prior to starting the tasks, he questioned the women as to their ability to complete the tasks. He called the women's perceived ability to cope *self-efficacy*. He found that the greater the women's perceived self-efficacy, the less stress they reported during the tasks and the lower their levels of stress hormones in their bloodstream during the task. Next, Bandura educated the women about spiders and had them repeat the tasks. After the instruction, the women reported greater self-efficacy, and they were able to complete the tasks without feeling stress and without a rise in their stress hormones. This was a remarkable and dramatic study. It showed that through education people can have a change of consciousness or attitude that enables them to have a healthy physiological response rather than an unhealthy one. Their change in consciousness resulted in a change in stress hormone levels, which affect blood pressure and immune function.

Other studies link attitude to illness in an even more direct way. The social psychologist Suzanne Kobasa studied the personality characteristics of a group of executives who experienced company upheaval and change. She found that some of the people became ill and others did not. She also found the healthy and unhealthy groups had distinct personality traits. She referred to the personality characteristics of the healthy group as *hardiness*. Kobasa found that hardiness consisted of three components: *control, commitment,* and *challenge.* Control involved a belief that one could influence the events taking place around oneself. Commitment involved a sense of taking an active role in one's life; it meant curiosity, a sense of purpose, and recognition of one's own value. Finally, challenge involved viewing change as stimulating rather than threatening. The hardy group approached stressful tasks with a sense of purpose and a belief in their abilities and the importance of the task.

The Israeli medical sociologist Aaron Antonovsky views coping skills not as a personality type but as a philosophy or world outlook. Working independently from Kobasa, Antonovsky defined a set of coping skills very similar to Kobasa's hardiness. The coping skills that result in health Antonovsky termed *a sense of coherence.* A sense of coherence is a way of looking at the world that gives people a sense of confidence that their environment is predictable. Antonovsky divides coherence into three parts: *comprehensibility, manageability,* and *meaningfulness.* Comprehensibility refers to the extent to which people see the world as making sense. It implies not that the world or an event is good or bad, but simply that it is understandable. Manageability refers to the extent to which people feel that they can meet life's demands. Meaningfulness is a measure of how much people care about a situation that confronts them. Antonovsky believes that when people have a strong sense of coherence, they see life events as opportunities rather than as threats, thereby minimizing the stress they feel and ultimately contributing to better health.

When people have positive attitudes and feel supported, they are more likely to stay well or to heal an illness if they do become sick. It is as if a positive mega-image sends a will-to-live message to each cell in the body. The mind acts as an organizing principle, coordinating information coming into the body. The brain is in continuous contact with all the cells of the body; in a person who has a basically positive attitude toward life, the messages from mind to body promote homeostasis, which brings about health and healing. Thus, we can make a remarkable generalization about mind/body processes, remarkable not only because it is profound, but because it is so simple. Positive states of mind promote healing. When the mind feels joy and delight, the body is more likely to heal. The implications of this statement are far-reaching. It essentially means that anything we can do to promote our happiness will also promote our health. The words "happiness" and "health" actually constitute a mantra, a phrase that, when repeated to oneself, gives a direction, in this case for healing.

Numerous studies have demonstrated the effects that support and attitude have on health. Basically, attitudes that promote happiness lead to health. Conversely, attitudes that prolong anxiety and despair can lead to illness. Attitudes act in conjunction with physical and environmental factors such as diet, exercise, genetic background, and disease organisms, and habits such as smoking and drinking. Positive attitudes that have been shown to enhance health include humor, caring, competence, self-efficacy, motivation, assertiveness, ability to express emotion, strong self-esteem, commitment, control, challenge, intimacy, social interaction, marital harmony, spiritual beliefs, a sense of belonging, connection with animals, flexibility, acceptance of change, optimism, comprehensibility, predictability, meaningfulness, and hope.

Negative attitudes that have been shown to promote illness include loneliness, depression, hopelessness, anxiety, fear, grief, lack of control, helplessness, suppressed anger, defensiveness, inability to express emotion, subservience, marital disruption, alienation, powerlessness, uncertainty, incomprehensibility, feelings of being victimized, and pessimism.

A classic study that demonstrated that a positive attitude can improve health dealt with arthritis management. Ann O'Leary of Stanford divided arthritis patients into two groups, one of which received an arthritis self-management course in addition to the normal medical treatment. The course was designed to help patients deal with pain and depression, as well as other physical symptoms. Patients were given information about nutrition and stress and were taught relaxation and physical exercises designed to strengthen their joints. The people who took the course reported a 28 percent reduction in pain, a 20 percent decrease in swelling, an 18 percent decrease in depression, and a 20 percent increase in perceived self-efficacy. O'Leary believes that those who improved had a positive outlook and felt a sense of control. A woman with cancer came to a workshop with feelings of hopelessness and depression. She was experiencing some pain and cried often during the first days of the workshop. After beginning imagery work, her mood became more cheerful. The sense that she was doing something positive changed her attitude. She stopped crying and started helping a man in the workshop who had great difficulty walking. Her pain disappeared, and her sense of humor emerged.

This study shows how important attitude, as well as physical factors, is to health and well-being. Love, happiness, joy and delight, and a sense of control free the body's healing abilities to work at their best, whereas depression, helplessness, and selfishness have a negative effect. The physiological mechanisms that underlie these effects are probably related to the effect of stress on the cardiovascular and immune systems. Joy and delight stimulate the immune system; helplessness and fear depress it.

A person's worldview or philosophy seems to act as an organizing force for the body. We can only speculate on why this is so. Why do we heal with joy and become ill in the face of sadness?

At the most basic level, the body is programmed to seek certain goals. These include survival and reproduction. Beyond that the goals become more psychological and spiritual in nature. Human beings seem to have an innate need to learn and to do things well—a desire for competence. This expresses itself in curiosity and the need to create. We also seem to have an innate desire to find order in the world, to understand how things work, and to make sense out of chaos.

In addition to seeking to understand their world, people have an inborn drive to find meaning in situations and to feel that their actions have an effect on the world they are a part of. Human beings also have an inborn tendency to form social relationships and to take care of each other. They have a need to love and be loved and to serve others. Many inborn needs have been addressed through religion. Through the ages, spiritual systems have sought to explain the origin and meaning of the phenomena that surround us and to define people's role in the universe. In the last several hundred years science has also attempted to explain physical phenomena. From the dawn of history myths have grown to try to explain what we see. When people believe that they understand the world around them, when they feel that they have a purpose and that their actions are important, something essential inside them is fulfilled.

Feelings of happiness, joy, and delight naturally accompany creativity and participation in the world; they reinforce our activities. Feelings of depression and anxiety surface when we aren't fulfilling our inborn needs. It's as if our inner center has images and goals for each of us that are reinforced by feelings of happiness, joy, and delight and are not reinforced by feelings of depression and loneliness. The human body is made of millions, even billions of cells working together at a high level of organization. The laws of physics tell us that it takes great energy to keep a complex system organized and active. The natural tendency is for systems to wind down or come apart unless energy is put into them. In that respect, each human body is a miracle. The mind provides the organizing principle. It corrals or gets together enough energy to maintain the system. At the most basic physical level, this involves getting sufficient food. At a more profound level, it involves creating a worldview that keeps a person motivated to survive. A worldview that involves actively and joyfully participating in the flow of the universe develops and releases tremendous energy. In this case, the energy is psychic. It may be crucial to keeping an organism alive.

At a deeper level we seem to be programmed to seek connection with the world around us, to see ourselves as one with other people, other animals, with nature itself. For many people there is a sense of themselves as part of, or one with, a greater force—something outside themselves. Throughout the ages, unity has been the goal of many religions. The purpose of meditation, prayer, ritual and devotion, and spiritual knowledge is to develop and make resonant this connection. Many Eastern religions believe that each person is actually one with the universe or with God and all other creatures but often does not see this because of his or her own "ignorance." Through reverie states and knowledge, the veils of ignorance can be lifted and the person can be freed to experience this reality.

One way of looking at positive emotions and health is that they reinforce our inborn need for interconnectedness or oneness. A well-known study by the Harvard researcher David McClelland emphasizes this relationship. McClelland found that when he showed a film of Mother Teresa tending the sick and dying to a group of college students, they had enhanced immune function, as evidenced by elevated levels of antibodies in their blood. The students experienced this rise whether or not they believed in Mother Teresa's work. McClelland believes that the concept of loving care exemplified by Mother Teresa reached the students at a subconscious level, naturally enhancing the response of their immune system. Similarly, researchers have found that relationships with pets seem to enhance people's immune function. The loving bonds that people establish with their pets have been shown to decrease blood pressure, lessen anxiety in cancer patients, and help relieve depression. Being happily married, maintaining close ties with children and friends, and joining groups and communities all act to increase people's sense of interconnectedness and to make us healthy. Conversely, loneliness, bereavement, lack of support, and withdrawal from people all serve to increase our feelings of separation and to slow healing or prevent it. From this point of view, stress is a symptom of separateness. When people feel anxious, fearful, or upset, they tense, tighten up, and withdraw into their body. This causes them to pull away from other people. When individuals feel loving and positive, they relax, open up, and go to the reverie state inside themselves, which expands their reality and causes them to reach out and connect with other people.

Stress results from our perception that something in our environment threatens our security. Initially it may only be someone's insult or negative comment. But the comment may act on aspects in us that were not validated as a child, thereby bringing up basic insecurities that make us contract and withdraw from the world. A large study done at Johns Hopkins University indicates that early childhood upbringing has an important effect on our health as adults. The psychiatrist Carolyn Thomas did a long-range prospective study on 1,300 medical students. She found that those who said they had positive relations with their parents during childhood, strong self-esteem, lack of depression, the ability to cope with stress, and an optimistic outlook tended to be healthy as adults, whereas students who reported poor relationships with their parents and others, ambivalent attitudes, and an attitude of personal avoidance tended to be less healthy as adults. In fact, these people had three to four times the risk of cancer as compared to the first group.

I believe that people can do a great deal toward making their attitude and worldview more positive. We do not have to be victims of our upbringing and repeat habitual negative reactions endlessly. We do not have to respond with fear and anxiety to situations that do not actually threaten us. We can learn to look for positive elements in situations, to look for love and oneness rather than negativity and separatism. And we have the reactions of our body and mind to guide us. When we feel prolonged stress and fear, we know we are off our path; when we feel joy and relaxation, we know we are following our bliss.

In this book I will help you create an attitude of healing. I will help you use guided imagery to change your worldview. Myths can play an important part in this process. One factor that contributes to the lack of a positive attitude is the absence of cultural myths that give people a reason for being. In tribal times cultures had stories that were believed to have come from the beginning of time. These stories told of the history of the world and the people's place in it. Often the stories actually stated that something that the people did was necessary for the world's creation and being. An example of such a myth has been related by Carl Jung. Jung recounted a conversation he had with Ochwiay Biano (Mountain Lake), a chief of the Taos Pueblo Indians. As they sat on the roof of the pueblo, 7,000 feet above sea level, looking out at the surrounding circle of mountains, Ochwiay Biano pointed at the sun and said with great emotion,

> Is not he who moves there our father? . . . We are a people who live on the roof of the world; we are the sons of Father Sun, and with our religion we daily help our father to go across the sky. We do this not only for ourselves, but for the whole world. If we were to cease practicing our religion, in ten years the sun would no longer rise. Then it would be night forever.[4]

For tribal peoples, myths like this give life profound purpose and meaning. Their lives become cosmologically meaningful, because their actions tie them to the movements of the universe. Jung believed that the mythic world from which such beliefs sprang was available to each of us and, in fact, was our home by right of birth. It is a home that we can reclaim with imagery.

For many people religion provides myths that give life meaning, linking their lives to a viewpoint that is larger than themselves. When people see the world around them as sacred, their perception of the world changes, transforming and altering all of their actions. However, for some people science has altered their view of religion so that they can no longer accept traditional myths at a level deep enough to transform their lives. For these people the spirit has gone out of the old myths, and their meaning is lost. Joseph Campbell believed that the basic myths of

Christianity and Judaism no longer apply to our age and that we await the birth of a new cultural myth. Many Christians such as the California theologian Matthew Fox are breathing life into their old symbols and applying them to ecology and world peace. Campbell believes that myths are expressed in symbols, that myths are universal truths, and that the symbols come from the tribe's collective experiences. Whereas the basic thought behind a myth is universal, the symbols and language of the myth must vary with the people involved. Campbell has said that the most important effect of a myth is to "waken and give guidance to the energies of life."[5] He believes that myths can reach a deep level of our consciousness, which actually wakes us up and fills us with tremendous energy. Myths also point us in a direction and help us channel our energy for a specific purpose. Myths work by directly addressing the body's feeling system—they do not have to be interpreted through logical thought. The universal voice of the myth speaks directly to our inner center. When a culture's central myths disappear or lose their meaning, people can lose their energy and direction.

I believe that some of the diseases common to this time in history reflect, in part, the loss of our central cultural myths. When we have lost the footprints of universal symbols, we lose much of the meaning of our life. This lack of meaning causes us to perceive the world less positively, which in turn results in stress. Fortunately, we have within us the ability to create or recognize new myths for us and for our times. The inner center can experience our myth and signal its presence with the feeling of "ah-h." This myth may be totally new, may be totally personal, or may relate to a religious belief structure. The most important factor is that the myth be a living one that can move our heart.

The creation or revivification of "our" myth involves a journey, a search. Most often throughout history, the search starts with suffering—either a tragedy, mental anguish, or physical illness. Carl Jung referred to the archetype for the suffering individual who becomes a shaman as "the wounded healer." Such suffering breaks down the habits and the assumptions by which we live. It alters the way we look at and deal with the world. In his suffering,

Buddha asked himself, "What are the symptoms of the world disease?" His answer was the First Noble Truth, "All life is sorrowful."[6] Out of suffering and the severing of habits comes separation, which is a retreat inward, deep into the land of reverie. The journey toward the inner center involves a series of encounters and experiences that, if we are successful, result in a new worldview and attitude, a rebirth to new life. Joseph Campbell views the mythological hero's journey as having three stages: *separation, initiation,* and *return.* The separation resulting from sorrow or illness causes us to yearn for a new worldview. The journey inward allows our inner center to balance our ego and heal the wounds from our childhood and our cultural conditioning. The rebirth is our coming back to life to see things in a new way. It is a transformation that brings light and clarity. Buddha's second question was, "Can a total cure be achieved?" The Second Noble Truth was "There is release from sorrow."[7] The Third Noble Truth described Buddha's view of health: "Release from sorrow is Nirvana," the extinction of egoism, which involves releasing individual desires and duties and the fear of death.[8] Now, this spiritual goal has important application to healing, for when we release ourselves from the anxieties and fears that result from unfulfilled desires, burdensome duties, and fear of dying, our soul is free to heal mind and body. In this larger sense, life itself is the journey, and healing can be a secondary effect of moving forward on a spiritual path. One metaphor for this is that each one of us has a path that makes special use of our skills. When our journey follows this path, we are constantly fulfilled. Every moment we do what is natural for us, we are in harmony with the creative forces of the universe. And we are helping to realize our higher self. The path we are describing is egoless in that it comes from our inner center and meshes with the needs of the world, not just our own needs.

All of us have difficulty staying true to our path. At points in our lives each one of us gets stuck, wanders from the path, or goes off in the wrong direction. When this happens, the universe sends us signals. One form these signals can take is discomfort or lack of ease. Stress is a perception that things are not quite right for us. Sometimes illness is associated with the discomfort, pain, and suffering of being off our path; sometimes illness is related to the stress engendered by losing our personal path. At other times illness that is predominantly genetic or environmental may not reflect our individual path at all. Nevertheless, illness can sometimes work to open up our awareness. An ancient Buddhist aphorism holds that illness is one of the things not to be avoided, because illness can act as a teacher. It causes us to stop and reevaluate where we are going. And it can be a positive force for getting us back on course; it can be the impetus for making small or large changes in our lives. Illness can teach us, even when it affects other people, friends, or loved ones. It causes us to reassess what is really important, really meaningful in our lives. Which is not to say that anyone wants to become ill or enjoys being ill. A man who had recovered from cancer responded to a questionnaire about his experiences by saying, "I've learned a lot from my illness, but it has been a giant pain in the ass, and I wouldn't wish it on anyone." Fortunately, people have the ability to move forward, to take what they have learned, and to leave pain and suffering behind.

It is important that the metaphor of illness as a messenger or teacher not be used to blame ourselves or others for becoming ill. First, we are all simply who we are. We are affected by our genetic background, our upbringing and conditioning, and the forces in the world around us. If all these forces beyond our control contribute to our *becoming* ill, the illness is not our "fault"; it is simply a result of a complex set of interactions. This does not mean that we cannot learn from the illness or act to improve the situation and perhaps bring about a cure. Many people consciously or subconsciously blame themselves or someone else for their illness. When people are told that attitude plays a causal role in illness, they often interpret this to mean that they are at fault. The goal of this model is not to assign blame or create guilt but to empower people to change themselves and their environment so as to promote health and happiness. In the end, the point is not *why* we become ill, but *how* we choose to deal with it. Just as the universe provides us with messages that tell us we're off the path, it provides us with messages to tell us when we're on the path. The messages that tell us we are expressing our inner self are joy and delight. The word "ah-h" is the expression of being on course. It conveys the feeling involved when we are following our path. A woman with a lymphoma became angry when she read a book that linked behavior to cancer. She believed strongly that her cancer was due to chemicals and not to anything in her attitude or actions. Because of this, she had initially rejected any psychological therapies in dealing with her illness. However, she was drawn to the idea of guided imagery. After her first exercises she realized that improving her present attitude helped her relinquish her anger and made her feel much better.

The Discussion

Basic images and attitudes keep people healthy and promote healing. When I work with people who are ill, I can see this all the time. People often come to a doctor frightened and in pain. A major part of healing is to turn this around, to replace fear with love and reassurance, to replace pain with comfort. The greatest effect of traveling inward is the spontaneous change in attitude that results. One woman that I worked with had multiple sclerosis. She came to the workshop not to deal with the MS, but to deal with fear of the future. She was an older, conservative person who worked in an office and had no previous imagery experiences. She participated in the workshop fully but did not say much about her experiences. Throughout the workshop, everyone could see and feel her increasing bravery and strength. As the workshop progressed, her face looked younger and younger, and she seemed to be less afraid of attempting new things. One beautiful day she decided to go to the beach. This meant leaving her motorized walker and crossing several hundred yards of boulders the size of melons. Holding a cane in each hand, she slowly manipulated herself across the boulders to the water's edge. The journey there and back took the whole afternoon and was magnificent to watch. I felt as if it was a symbol of her ability to go anywhere. The change in her attitude preceded her healing. The attitude change need only be a general "I can do it." It comes from looking around and seeing things as sacred. From beauty come images of power and support.

There are many exercises that people can do to encourage positive attitudes and create and hold positive mega-images. The first exercise focuses on picturing life events and imagining how changing your basic attitudes would affect them. The idea is to imagine an event clearly and see how the event would change with different attitudes. During the imagery, focus on how your body feels as you try out these changes. The theme of this exercise is that you can learn to change your attitudes and have much greater control over attitudes and emotions than you realize.

The second exercise deals with a personal myth. A myth that a person can live by is a helper on the journey. It frees our healing energies and promotes a positive attitude by increasing a sense of meaningfulness, comprehensibility, and coherence. Myths work at deep levels that are below the level of words. In this chapter we will do a brief exercise to start us on our way toward evolving a personal myth.

Our exercise starts with a shamanic initiation. Such initiation rituals traditionally involved a systematic stripping away of the old so that the new can emerge. The exercise then moves to a vision in which we glimpse our own creation myth; it ends by having us examine our special gifts in order to clarify our place in the creative universe. The process of building a myth is a long and active one. It takes time and it takes work. For most of us the process is lifelong. This exercise is one way of starting out, even though the process is highly individual.

In my experience this is a powerful exercise. People enjoy it and are changed by it. Many people experience these visions themselves during unguided imagery journeys brought about by drumming or music. The experience of being reduced to the essence and then rebuilding oneself must be profound and deep. The changes it echoes are far below consciousness. It takes time for the effects to be felt and understood, but in my experience people are transformed by it. The exercise can also be disturbing, but proceed with it and you will be all right.

The Exercises

Exercise 5—Changing Attitudes: Empowerment.

Find a comfortable space where you will not be disturbed. Sit or lie down with your legs uncrossed, your arms at your sides or resting on your abdomen. Loosen any tight or constricting clothing. Close your eyes. Begin by inhaling slowly and deeply through your nostrils. Let the breath out through your nose slowly and completely. Continue breathing in this manner, allowing your abdomen to rise as you inhale and fall as you exhale. As you breathe allow yourself to relax.

Now picture in your mind a recent event in which you were required to adapt or make changes in your life. It may be an event involving your work, family life, or medical treatment. First allow the event itself to come to mind, and once you recognize it, let it start to become real. Feel yourself entering the scene, and look around you and see what it's like. Feel the floor under your feet, smell the air, and listen to the voices of the people around you. Allow the event to take place in your mind, and see and feel as many details as you can. As the event occurs be particularly aware of your attitudes and any body sensations of pleasure, relaxation, tension, or discomfort. Also be aware of feelings such as happiness, joy, anxiety, or fear. Simply experience these sensations; don't become attached to them or make judgments about them. When you become aware of the sensations, note them in your mind but go on with the event.

Now imagine that the same event takes place but the outcome is not as positive. Mentally create a whole new scenario in which many of the particulars turn out worse for you. Again, see, feel, and hear the scene in detail, and be aware of your attitudes and feelings. Now picture the scene a third time. This time, picture it in a way that the outcome is much better. Use all your senses to make the scene real, and watch how your attitudes change and your body reacts to this positive scene.

Imagine that at some time prior to the event you could create new basic images and attitudes. First, imagine that your ability to handle the particular event increases markedly. Imagine that you increase your confidence by increasing your preparation, skills, or belief in yourself. Next, ask yourself what you can do to learn and benefit from the event. What can you get out of it at a basic level? How can the event become more of a challenge? Think of at least one thing in the event that is interesting and exciting and would enrich your life. Next, ask yourself how important the event is to your life. Will it help make your life or the lives of others better? How can you increase the event's meaningfulness and your commitment to the event's outcome? Find at least one thing in the event that is important to you. Finally, ask yourself what specific things you can do to affect the event's outcome. How can you increase your control in this situation? Find at least one thing that you can do, no matter how small, that will change the course of the event.

Now allow the event to occur again in your mind. This time try to bring your ideas for increasing self-confidence, challenge, commitment, and control to the situation. As the event unfolds, use your ideas to make the scene increasingly positive. Incorporate any new ideas that come to you, and allow the scene to become richer and more elaborate.

Rest for a minute; breathe in deeply through your nose and let the breath out slowly. Let your abdomen rise and fall. Let yourself relax, and continue breathing in and out deeply. Let any feelings of tingling or warmth increase. Now imagine that you are in a secure, peaceful space. Imagine that feelings of encouragement and acceptance flow into you. Remember times in your life when people have supported you and validated you. Let the memories become real and positive feelings increase in your body. Now imagine that you can feel the flow of the universe around you, feel its power and movement. Realize that you are a part of this process and that what you do helps the universe grow. Picture your actions as part of the creative flow of the world. Imagine that what you do is full of life and beauty and that it makes the world a better place. Trust in the process and help it along.

When you wish to return to your everyday state, gently move your feet and count slowly from one to three. You will return to your everyday state relaxed and full of energy. Your body will feel as if it is in a comfortable, healing space. Each time you do this exercise you will relax more deeply and more easily. The feelings of relaxation will deepen, and the whole exercise will become more and more pleasurable.

This exercise is used in different forms by many therapists working with attitude. The results of the exercise just happen. People feel that they have a greater understanding of the role that attitude plays in their life. The exercise demonstrates how control, commitment, and challenge are involved in outcome. Even though it takes place in our imagination, it affects our choices in future events. The exercise also points out how success-oriented we are.

The other exercises in the book deal with more spiritual concerns. The next exercise takes you to a very different space. Before beginning it, rest or go for a walk and let the previous exercise drift away.

Exercise 6—Toward a Personal Myth.

Find a comfortable space where you will not be disturbed. Sit or lie down with your legs uncrossed, your arms at your sides or resting on your abdomen. Loosen any tight or constricting clothing. Close your eyes. Begin by inhaling slowly and deeply through your nostrils. Let the breath out through your nose slowly and completely. Continue breathing in this manner, allowing your abdomen to rise as you inhale and fall as you exhale. As you breathe allow yourself to relax.

Allow the feelings of relaxation to spread over your body. Allow your feet to relax. Allow your legs to relax, and let your muscles lengthen. Let the relaxation spread up to your pelvic area. Continue to breathe deeply. With each breath, your body will become more and more relaxed. Allow any worries or anxieties that you have to drift off. Release them—you don't need them here. Now let your abdomen and chest relax. Let the relaxation spread to your upper arms and down to your fingers. Notice the feeling of tingling in your fingers and let it increase. Let the tingling spread throughout your body, and relax even more deeply. Now let your neck relax, and let your head relax.

Now deepen the relaxation by counting from ten to one as you breathe in and out. On the first breath, as you inhale, say to yourself, "Ten," and as you exhale say, "Deeply relaxed." With the next breath, as you inhale say, "Nine" and as you exhale, "Deeply relaxed." Inhale: "Eight . . . even more relaxed." Continue counting and breathing until you reach one.

You are now at a deeper and more relaxed level, a level at which time and space are different. At this level you can see and imagine things clearly. Rest a moment and breathe deeply. Imagine that you are on a path in a forest at dusk. It is warm, and you are wearing lightweight clothes. You are walking down a path. In front of you and behind you are many others, walking the same path. The path winds gently downward, crosses a tiny stream with small rocks you can step on to cross, and climbs slowly up a hill. As you walk it gets darker. Feel the soft earth under your feet and hear the noises of the forest around you. As you walk feel the warm air on your face and arms. You feel excited because you know that this is the day of your initiation. You don't know what will happen to you, but you trust the elders.

The path leaves the forest and enters a clearing. There is a circle about seventy feet in diameter. It is now dark. All of the people sit around the edge of the circle. Now you feel hands behind you lifting you up from the sitting position in the circle. It is the elders, your teachers tapping you to begin. You stand and they take you into the forest and guide you to a stone. It is the ceremonial stone for shamanic initiation used by many who have gone before you. You lay on the stone and close your eyes.

The figures reach their hands toward you, and your body starts to come apart. Let your body come apart, let it separate. Each person can let it come apart to a different point. If at any time this process feels uncomfortable, stop and rest and go back. This exercise is safe; if you are comfortable you can go as far as you wish. First your skin comes off, then your muscles. Only your skeleton is left on the table. Finally your skeleton starts to break apart. The arm bones come off, the leg bones come off, the ribs come off, the skull comes off. The spine comes apart. Finally one vertebra is all that is left on the stone. The vertebra starts to glow; it glows bluish white. It gets brighter. The rock platform now begins to change; it develops a curve in the center and begins to resemble half an eggshell. Your consciousness remains in the eggshell for a long time.

A figure appears in the background. It is larger than the other figures. It stretches its hand out toward your vertebra. You sense that it is full of goodness. Mysteriously the outlines of a new body start to appear out of nowhere. They are filmy and smokelike but have the size and shape of your old body. This new body becomes more real but is still transparent, full of air, and made of tiny dots of light. The body becomes more and more solid, more and more dense. Although it is still made of light, the dense material begins to predominate. The new body feels wonderful. It is incredibly strong and calm. The figure touches your new hand. You get up from the slab and stand. The energy in your new body is immense. As you start walking with the figure you are using only a tiny bit of your new body's power.

The figure leads you out of the cave onto a path. Your body becomes denser and denser as you walk. You can see other figures with new bodies, and their guardians, walking in front of you and behind you. You step up on a bridge that arches upward and enters a sphere. The sphere is made of smoky gray light and is floating. You cross the bridge and enter the sphere. The figure seats you in the center of the sphere, then starts to speak. It tells you that the sphere is a special image-producing device of your people. It is the place where people are able to see their own myth and that of their people: it is a myth finder. The symbols of the myth appear as images or thoughts inside the sphere. They may appear toward the sphere's edges or float in the center. The sphere itself has a wonderful half-light quality, like the moments before dawn. The edges of the sphere are diffuse; it is like looking into a dense white fog.

First the myth finder will reveal to you your image of the beginning of the universe. Look around the sphere, and when something begins to form in the fog, focus on it. It may be an image of a horizon, of a figure, or of a light. Let the images float. Let the story unfold in your mind. Do not be concerned if the images are unclear or incomplete; you can return to the myth finder any time to see more.

Now let the myth finder reveal to you images about the beginning of the earth. As images emerge from the fog, focus on them. You may see a ball, rocks and mountains, fire or water. Let the images float. Let the events unfold in your mind. Now invite images that reveal the beginnings of the animal world and of people. Let the first people come alive; hear their story. Now let yourself see the story of your own ancestors. Let them come alive. Listen to their story. Ask them why they are here, what their purpose is in this world, what their goals are for the future. Now allow the images in the sphere to disappear.

Now look toward the edges of the sphere, into the fog, and search for images of joy from your childhood and teenage years. If negative images arise, turn them aside. Allow images to form of what you most liked doing throughout your childhood. They may be images of playing, working at hobbies, participating in sports, or working in school. Spend time with each of these images; feel the enjoyment that each of these scenes holds. Now let the scene move slowly forward in time. Let the images deal with things you have enjoyed doing as an adult. Again, you may see images relating to hobbies or interests, your job or family, organizations or religious groups to which you belong. Spend time with each of these images; feel the enjoyment that each of them brings. Now let images move even further forward in time. Allow images to emerge from the fog that concern scenes of joy from your future. Again, they may relate to work, family, hobbies, religion, or other aspects of your life. Spend time with these scenes and feel the joy of them. Now allow images to emerge of the special gifts you have. See yourself—past, present, or future—doing what you do best. Feel the feelings of pride and love that occur when you use your gifts to their utmost.

Now allow all the images of joy and delight from your past, present, and future to come together and tell a story. Look at all of your moments of joy and delight and the special gifts you have as pieces of your personal myth. Now allow the guardian who brought you to the sphere to appear beside you. Let the images and story of your reason for being here come to your consciousness now. You may see lots of loose images or a group of images that are linked together, or you may hear the story from your guardian. Don't be concerned if the story isn't clear to you now. You can return to the sphere at any time. Some people never see the story in its entirety; rather, they feel it unfold as bliss throughout their lives.

Allow yourself to rest in the sphere as long as you wish. Let the energy from the light of the sphere merge with the energy from your new body. Let this energy make you feel vibrant and whole. Stay there as long as you wish. When you are ready to return to your usual state of consciousness, count slowly from one to three and gently move some part of your body. Rest for a while in this state. Realize that you can return whenever you wish and that each time it will be easier and the feelings stronger. Open your eyes when you wish to do so.

Most people find this exercise to be an unusual experience. Some people have described it as moving and exciting, even scary; others say they find it deeply relaxing. I've found the imagery of being taken apart and reduced to one's essence and then reformed anew to be basic and powerful. Even if people do not feel much during the exercise, the experience seems to be a catalyst for change. Simply experiencing this symbolic rebirth seems to prepare a person for new ideas and new directions for growth. It's like preparing the ground for new seeds. One woman, a physical therapist, saw images of herself being taken apart and almost disappearing completely, and felt a new body being created for her. She then saw a circle of shamanic figures working on her new body and giving it healing powers. After the exercise, she felt a new power in herself, and she developed a deep interest in ritual and started to incorporate many new routines and practices into her physical therapy work. For her, the exercise opened up a whole new area of her personality, both in terms of herself and her own interests and in terms of her work and her patients. Up to then, her work and her interests had been primarily physical; now they became much more spiritual. A child psychologist who did this exercise saw a shiny pearl after her body had been reduced to its essence. The preciousness and beauty of that image gave her a powerful sense of her own purity and made her feel valued.

Some people who do the exercise are bothered by the concept that their experience grows out of my suggestions and is therefore not completely their own. Images come from many sources. In traditional cultures, imagery is taught by tribal elders and shamans and is deeply embedded in the culture. The youth in these cultures will have been given suggestions since childhood concerning their vision quest and initiation. The images they see do not come out of the air. Likewise, in our culture, images come from cultural experiences such as reading books, seeing movies, going to lectures, or watching television shows. Events that you are attracted to in the outer world become symbols of change in the inner world. Your perceptions of the outer world reflect your inner world. Thus inner images often relate to seemingly mundane experiences in the outer world. But this makes them no less powerful or effective.

Sometimes people worry because they feel as if they are "making up" the images that they experience in the exercise. They believe that the images should feel as if they are coming from somewhere else. Because we see the images in our mind, they feel like thoughts, and they naturally feel as if we're creating them. As we glimpse them coming from our inner center, we catch them and flesh them out. This process definitely has some of the feelings of creating images or making them up. When I work with people, I emphasize the point that the feeling of making things up is the *correct* feeling. Moreover, I advise people to go with that feeling and let an element of making it up merge with the images that come from inside.

Finally, with this exercise, most people experience images of a creation myth that are similar to, or tied to, material they have learned from science and religion. One man in a workshop saw an image of the universe expanding and felt himself riding a light beam moving toward the edge of space. He felt a timeless connection with the world around him, felt that he was the same as the rest of the world. He felt that he understood the Hindu aphorism "I am that." At the same time he felt guilty that his imagery involved the scientific theory of the expanding universe that he had learned in college. Again, the source of our images doesn't take away from their power. In many ways the strongest images derive from our cultural inheritance. In all these exercises, do not censor your images; honor them. The most profound effects of the exercises take place below the level of conscious thought.

4

Inner Guides:
Helping Figures

Inner guides are a major force in my life. Since I first read about their existence, I have been intuitively interested in them, and from the time that I met the first of my own guides and began using a guide in my life, I've found guides to be one of my major interests. At this point I would almost say that inner guides are my specialty. When I teach workshops I focus on the concept of inner guides, and when I work with cancer patients, I work with inner guides as well as imagery. The goal of this chapter is to allow people who are interested in guides to learn more about them, meet them, and begin to work with them.

Because we encounter the guide in a reverie state, experience makes it real. Meeting and using a guide is a life experience. The feelings that surround the use of a guide really define guides and give us trust in them, more than theory and explanation do. Guides are a basic tool for getting in touch with the inner center. In this way I see guides as a primary healing tool. In a real sense, guides are the voice of the inner center. Their information comes from the inner world; they are a major way that the personality, or ego, can have an active dialogue with the inner center.

Over the years my understanding of guides has changed. At present I see the guide as equal in importance to the source of the guide's information. The guide is the voice of the inner center, and that knowledge and understanding are as important as the guide itself. The inner center also speaks to us through dreams, symbols, intuitive flashes, creative ideas, and feelings of bliss. Through guides, the inner center speaks to us more directly. In addition, guides make it possible for us to ask questions and direct the subject of our dialogue. Imagine that your inner center is a huge source of energy and information. A guide is a way to bring some of this material directly to consciousness.

Because the guide is so valuable, it is not surprising that it has been a basic tool of mankind for thousands of years. Many tribal cultures and religions have used guides throughout history for problem solving, healing, and the pursuit of spiritual oneness. Since guides are a concept that is foreign to our culture, a discussion of the history of guides should help make you more comfortable with the concept and the exercises that involve guides. I include historical, religious, and psychological explanations about guides, encompassing many different cultural traditions. I hope that after reading this material you will feel more at ease with the concept and more readily meet a guide of your own.

The first figure to actively use guides was the shaman. Guides have always been basic to shamanic healing. The shaman depends on personal power and an ability to travel in the inner world and interact with spirits to heal. Shamans believe that guardians and helping spirits give people power and protect them in the inner world. The anthropologist Ruth Benedict has observed that shamanism is built around the "vision–guardian spirit complex." Guardian spirits of shamans have been referred to by many terms in anthropological literature. They are referred to as "helping spirits" by Siberian shamans, "nagual" by Mexican and Guatemalan shamans, and "assistant totems" by Australian shamans. In shamanic healing, the guardian spirit is often seen as a power animal. During a healing, the shaman often becomes one with the guardian spirit.

Many American Indian tribes believe that all people have guardian spirits, whether or not they are shamans and whether or not the people can see their spirits. Traditionally in North American Indian tribes people met their guardian spirit after a vision quest. Such a quest involved going into the wilderness, enduring hardships, and meditating. South American shamans often used psychoactive drugs to help people meet their guardian spirit. Some Indian tribes, such as the Chumash of California, believed that a person did not become an adult until he or she met a guardian, and that a person could not live a normal life without one.

In traditional shamanism, there are two types of guardian spirits: *helping spirits,* which are also called *familiars* or *assistants,* and *tutelary spirits,* which are much more powerful and are considered to be semidivine. The shamans control their helper spirits but pray to the tutelary spirits, over which they have no control. Both types of spirits can be seen and talked to by more than one person. Also, shamans generally have more than one helping spirit. The names, forms, and numbers of spirits vary from region to region. The majority of helping spirits have animal forms.

An example of the complexity of a shaman's relationship with the spirits is given by the history-of-religions scholar Mircea Eliade in his classic work *Shamanism.* He describes a Siberian shaman who has seven helping spirits and three tutelary spirits. The latter consist of a spirit of a head that defends him during his journeys, a spirit of a bear that accompanies him on descents to the underworld, and a spirit of a gray horse that he rides on ascents to the sky. The Siberian tutelary spirits include lords of the sea and the wind. Often power animals can appear in human form and reveal their identity to the shaman. For many, any object can become a source of power or a guardian spirit: water, the sun, people, bones or hair or teeth of the dead, the sky, people's genital organs, even the directions of the compass. Eliade concludes that

> guardian spirits and mythical animal helpers are not a specific and exclusive characteristic of shamanism. These tutelary and helping spirits are collected almost anywhere in the entire cosmos, and they are accessible to any individual who is willing to undergo certain ordeals to obtain them. This means that everywhere in the cosmos archaic man recognizes a source of the magico-religious sacred, that any fragment of the cosmos can give rise to a hierophany, in

accordance with the dialectic of the sacred. What differentiates a shaman from any other in the clan is not his possessing a power or a guardian spirit, but his ecstatic experience. But as we have already seen, and shall see even more fully later, guardian or helping spirits are not the direct authors of this ecstatic experience. They are only the messengers of the divine being or the assistants in an experience that implies many other presences besides theirs.[1]

I interpret Eliade to mean that anyone who wants a helping spirit can get one, with work, and that he believes that spirits help bring the sacred to life.

Another major use of guides developed in Eastern thought. East Indian religions that use imagery have long recognized that forces of universal thought such as wisdom and compassion appear to meditators in embodied form. Thus people who meditate see and talk to deities that appear to them during specific imagery exercises. In Tantric Buddhism a lama assigns a student to meditate on a specific deity that is called a *yidam*. These yidams appear to the meditator as external beings. Buddhists are taught to realize that the yidam is the embodiment of a reality present at deeper levels of their mind, that these figures are, at the same time, emanations of their own mind and emanations of the ultimate reality. The purpose of the yidam is to transform the meditator and bring him or her closer to enlightenment. In more advanced exercises, meditators become one with the yidam, that is, they identify with the yidam, and make offerings to the yidam throughout the day. The yidam is another example of a paradox: the yidam is seen by the meditator as a real object, but it is also seen as a creation of the person's mind. The lamas believe that when a person visualizes a yidam, he or she manifests the internal world and brings it out into the external world. At the same time the person brings the external into the internal world. This process ultimately breaks a person free of the bounds of internal and external. Internal and external become one; the paradox is resolved.

.   .   .

Our examination of guides now moves to the realm of the twentieth-century psychologist. Carl Jung, who was a pioneer in exploring the unconscious, also devoted great study to the uses and values of guides. After parting ways with Freud, Jung found himself greatly disoriented. He had learned much about the unconscious but had not yet found his own footing. He asked himself what myth he lived in, and in thinking about it, he realized he did not have one. So he allowed his unconscious to become his guide and began to examine his dreams. The symbols in his dreams were so complicated that he was forced to acknowledge his own ignorance and to do whatever occurred to him. He consciously made a decision to follow his unconscious. One day while traveling on a train, Jung had a vision of a monstrous flood covering Europe. When the vision reappeared a second time, an inner voice spoke to him and told him the vision was real. The visions were precognitions of World War I, which would start in less than a year. But the experience of the truth of these visions profoundly shocked Jung, and he decided to devote himself to translating emotions into images. Jung had believed that he was pursuing a scientific experiment in which he voluntarily confronted his unconscious. Later, in looking back on this period, he felt more as if it was an experiment being conducted on him. After much deliberation he realized that he had to let himself drop into his unconscious and stop resisting it. On September 12, 1913, Jung let himself drop.

> Suddenly it was as though the ground literally gave way beneath my feet, and I plunged down into the dark depths. I could not fend off a feeling of panic. But then, abruptly, at not too great a depth, I landed on my feet in a soft, sticky mass. I felt great relief, although I was apparently in complete darkness. After a while my eyes grew accustomed to the gloom, which was rather like a deep twilight. Before me was the entrance to a dark cave, in which stood a dwarf with a leathery skin, as if he were mummified.[2]

The vision goes on in detail, and Jung was stunned by it.

Then Jung began to use conscious tools to bring the visions on.

In order to seize hold of the fantasies I frequently imagined a steep descent. I even made several attempts to get to the very bottom. The first time I reached, as it were, the depth of about a thousand feet; the next time I found myself at the edge of a cosmic abyss. It was like a voyage to the moon or a descent into empty space. First came the image of a crater, and I had the feeling that I was in the land of the dead. The atmosphere was that of the other world. Near the steep slope of rock I caught sight of two figures, an old man with a white beard and a beautiful young girl. I summoned up my courage and approached them as though they were real people, and listened attentively to what they told me. The old man explained that he was Elijah, and that gave me a shock.[3]

Jung continued his explorations of the unconscious, and after this exercise he met many inner figures. After many experiences in the inner realm, Jung found that the Elijah figure changed into an Egyptian-Greek wise old man whose name was Philemon. To Jung, Philemon represented superior insight. In his imagery, Jung walked up and down in a garden and asked the old man questions. Jung felt that Philemon was an inner teacher or guru, a *psychagogue*. He thought a great deal about what these inner figures were and developed a theory for what they represented:

Philemon and other figures of my fantasy brought home to me the crucial insight that there are things in the psyche that I do not produce, but which produce themselves and have their own life. Philemon represented a force which was not myself. In my fantasies I held conversations with him, and he said things which I had not consciously thought. For I observed clearly that it was he who spoke, not I. He said I treated thoughts as if I generated them myself, but in his view thoughts were like animals in the forest, or people in a room, or birds in the air, and added, "If you should see people in a room, you would not think that you had made those people, or that you were responsible for them." It was he who taught me psychic objectivity, the reality of the psyche. . . . I understood that there is something in me which can say things that I do not know and do not intend. . . . Psychologically, Philemon represented superior insight. He was a mysterious figure to me. At times he seemed to me quite real, as if he were a living personality.[4]

Jung believed that inner figures were personifications of unconscious content. The mind personified these inner concepts, Jung thought, because they truly had a degree of autonomy and identity of their own. Eventually Jung recorded six volumes of his fantasies, elaborately worded and written in calligraphy. Jung commented that the wording was elaborate because he found that archetypes often speak in rhetorical or grandiloquent language. The figures were so vivid that Jung recorded many of them in pictures. Jung believed that the information came to him in various ways. Sometimes he heard it with his ears, sometimes he felt as if his tongue were speaking it, sometimes he felt it in his body, and sometimes he actually heard himself whispering it.

Sometimes Jung was afraid that the fantasies would take him over. At one point Jung and even his family believed that objects in his house were being moved and that his whole house was full of spirits. The spirits seemed to disappear as soon as he wrote down the fantasies in which they had appeared. During these scary periods he felt that his family and his professional work were a support to him. He would say to himself, "I have a medical diploma from a Swiss university, I must help my patients, I have a wife and five children, I live at 228 in Seestrasse in Kushnacht."[5] His family and profession guaranteed him a normal life in his mind. Jung believed that not only was it important to allow inner images to arise and be seen, but it was important to allow them to change his life. That is, we are ethically bound to make use of the information that we receive from our unconscious. In other words, people have to act in the outer world on the basis of their understanding of information from the inner world. External actions are an essential part of the process. For Jung, his work was the way he used inner material in the outer world. For a person who is ill, making lifestyle changes represents the use of inner material in the outer world.

I am always amazed by how many people in our scientific

culture are attracted to these models of inner guides. Almost everyone can find some point of reference that is familiar or that speaks to them. I have included details because in my experience, the details add to the richness of people's experiences. The experiences of patients and workshop participants are incredibly similar to experiences of shamans, monks, and psychologists, and many of the details in these experiences are actually universal. Certainly Carl Jung's experiences of ascent and descent and his reaching for grounding are common to almost everyone.

Having briefly discussed the history of guides from shamanic, spiritual, and psychological viewpoints, we will now address practical concerns that are useful in meeting your own guide. The information in this next section comes from my experiences using guides with patients and from my experiences with my own guides. I've used guides in the treatment of people in a family practice, and I've used them with people who have cancer, AIDS, and other life-threatening illnesses. I have taught the technique to health professionals who wanted to use imagery in their practice, and I have taught it to people in workshops and retreats who were interested in inner work. The material in this chapter is based on all of their experiences. For you, like them, the goal is experience. Only by actually spending time with a guide can the concept become useful and real. As I've said earlier, guides are basic tools for personal growth and healing. A guide is a voice from the inner center that gives us information beyond the reach of our conscious thought that can help to balance and heal us. My own personal belief is that guides are personifications of symbols from our inner center, yet they are real beings in the reverie space. Guides also resolve the paradox of inner and outer. Because our inner center is real and is connected to the source, the guide can be both a personification of mind and a figure outside our mind.

My theories about guides are interesting to me, but they are not necessary for a reader attempting to find a guide. Theory is secondary to experience; the importance of guides lies in their usefulness. To hammer in a nail, it is not necessary to know who invented the hammer and whether that concept came from a person or from an idea floating in space. So it is with guides. However, theory is important in one regard. To begin to use a guide you need a certain degree of trust. In shamanic or spiritual work, that trust comes from faith in the shaman or guru and from having been raised in a culture that believes in spirits or gods. For Carl Jung, trust came from his lifelong belief in the unconscious and the mystical and from validation of his beliefs through his work with patients.

Most readers of this book will likely begin building their trust by linking it to the closest belief system they have. That trust may be based on the experience of physicians using guides; it may come from shamanic or mystical historicity; or it may come from a person's own way of looking at the world, whether it be a psychological view of the unconscious or a spiritual view of a divine force. A person's own view of what a guide is will be useful because it lays a groundwork for trust.

What are guides used for? Basically guides are a way of posing questions to our inner center. So their primary use becomes self-balancing, because the inner center, almost by definition, is homeostatic. First, the inner center is self-balancing in that it puts people's actions in harmony with their path. Second, the inner center balances the complicated workings of the body. Thus the inner center knows a person's path and is in control of the body's immune and autonomic nervous systems. It has intimate knowledge of the condition and workings of the body. In a sense, it actually possesses the health information of the body and controls the body's healing tools. So the voice of the inner center is a precious link to information that is often inaccessible to us consciously.

All of this means that the guide can be used as an oracle. If asked, guides can provide answers concerning a person's personal myth, meaning, and purpose. To use a metaphor of Larry LeShan's, guides can help people find their own song. Guides can provide answers that contain creative ideas and, in this way, function as a muse that helps to bring artwork and inventions into the outer world. Guides can provide practical information about job and family concerns, and they can offer advice on what a person can do to heal an illness. Guides can help a sick person work out personal healing advice dealing with nutrition, exercise, stress reduction, and using or choosing medical therapies. Each person has his or her own healing path, and a guide can help the individual discern that path. In all work with guides, the assumption is that the information comes from a source deeper than the person's ego or culturally determined "oughts" and "shoulds." The answers that come from a guide take a lot of pressure off the ego or personality in that they suggest decisions that seem to come from outside. People who use a guide feel as if they have help and do not have to make their decisions alone.

A major use of a guide, therefore, is as a support system. A guide offers companionship and makes a person feel less lonely, less isolated. This is a characteristic of all reverie experiences because they tie people to something outside themselves. At a very deep level, all inner centers and all guides are linked together. Thus the more that people function in a reverie state, the more connected they feel in the outer world.

The last use of a guide is in balancing the world. Not only are all guides connected to one another, but they are connected to the guide of the living earth. The astrophysicist James Lovelock has stated in the Gaia hypothesis that the earth behaves as if it were a living creature, that is, it has the characteristics of a living system in that it can regulate its temperature, amount of oxygen, degree of oceanic salinity, and so on. I also believe that the earth has an inner center, spirit, or soul and has inner guides. As unusual as this sounds, it is a timeless concept. Tribal cultures have always recognized and dealt with earth spirits, as well as spirits of the sun and moon. The people felt that these spirits were alive and that their interchanges with the spirits were necessary for their personal survival and for that of the earth. Working with a guide puts people more in touch with the spirit of the earth and makes our decisions more likely to be in harmony with the earth. In these times, when the earth is at hazard, contact with its inner center may actually be crucial for our survival.

What does a guide experience feel like? It feels like a conversation with a part of oneself. The figure with whom you're conversing tends to behave like a separate person. It has its own voice, its own speaking style (perhaps even an accent), its own vocabulary, tone, and cadence. What it says will often be surprising. When you hear yourself having a conversation with a guide, your own voice will sound and feel like you. When you talk to the guide, you consciously choose your words and thoughts, but the guide's responses feel different. You tend to listen to them, and the guide's answers tend to flow automatically, but you don't have as much of a feeling of choosing the words. You can recognize your guide's voice somewhat as you recognize a friend's voice on the telephone. The voice has its own characteristics and sounds as if it's coming from somewhere else. Yet at the same time, because it's coming through your mind, you may have the feeling that you're making the whole thing up. In a sense, you are, but the part of you making it up is deeper than the part of you that is responding. During a talk with an inner guide you feel a little different than usual. Those feelings are the feelings of a reverie state. You are calm and relaxed, space is expanded, time changes, your body expands, and generally there's a feeling of depth to the whole experience.

What types of guides are there? I believe that guides are symbols of parts of our inner center. So the forms that guides come in are shaped by our own inner symbols. I have found that every person has many guides who have different purposes and varied roles to play. The symbol that a guide manifests itself through is dependent on the purpose and role of the guide as well as our own personality and the time and place in which we live. Guides can manifest themselves as different symbols when necessary, that is, as whatever we are most attuned to and can most easily deal with. I believe that the shapes we project onto guides are less important than what the guide stands for. The guide is the embodiment of a concept and is thus universal. The guide's shape is less general and more particular to the individual.

Guides most often manifest as figures. I refer to this type of inner guide as a *spirit guide.* Usually they are human, women and men of the time we live in. However, they also can be from other times in history and can be larger than life or mythological, as in the case of Jung's Philemon. The figures can also be celestial or godlike, resembling biblical or spiritual figures or angels. In some cases guides are living people or people we've known in the past. There are even stories of people getting a guide whom they later met in real life. Probably the reason guides appear most often as figures is that we are used to having conversations with people. Also, I believe that the guises that guides appear in have much to do with the exercises that are used to teach people to meet their guide. Most exercises suggest that the guide will be a figure. Indeed, figures are easier for most people to deal with as guides.

The second most common form of guide is an animal. This was the most common type in shamanic and Native American cultures. Often the guides were magical animals or spirit animals, magical in the sense that they could talk and had knowledge of human concerns. Sometimes animal guides don't speak but communicate through other means, such as thoughts, body sensations, or more primitive feelings. These animals resemble the power animals that shamans use. They are much more likely to appear after suggestions in shamanic-type initiation exercises.

Another type of guide involves a less specific presence. This may be an area of light, a sound, a plant, an energy field, a cloud, or a voice that has no body. Some people do not see or hear their guide in the usual ways but are aware of presences that act as guides. This brings us to the way guides communicate. Some people see the guide, hear its voice, and can even touch and smell the guide; some people hear the guide but don't see it. Other people feel the guide in their body as energy. Some people get thoughts or visions that feel as if they come from their guide. Other people get emotions or bodily feelings, such as a sudden feeling of ease or confidence. Among the wide variety of guide experiences, the common feature that all of them share is that the information feels as if it is coming from outside.

I have found that people can have more than one guide and more than one type of guide. I also believe that the guide's form and appearance is changeable, although the underlying concept remains the same. Each type of guide fulfills a specific purpose or goal in a person's growth. One may have information about people's creative enterprises or work and may even function as a muse that dictates ideas to them; another may have expertise about personal relationships with a spouse or children; others may be spiritual advisers and deal primarily with religious concerns. In terms of this book, some guides are specifically healers or are knowledgeable about healing.

Carl Jung, who encountered many figures in his inner explorations, believed that guides are personifications or *archetypes,* basic concepts or symbols that are experienced universally, both by people in different cultures and by people of different times. For Jung, his Elijah/Philemon figure represented *logos,* or intelligence/knowledge, and his Salome figure represented the erotic character of an inner female figure that he termed the *anima.* Given that inner figures appear to be personifications of universal concepts, a figure's expertise relates to what it personifies. In other words, a wise old man has his own information to impart, different from that of a beautiful young girl. Individual guides do not have answers to all questions. In fact, they often don't know a great deal outside of their area of expertise. A guide concerned with healing may not have much advice about creativity or job concerns. It is also interesting that people usually get the type of guide that they need or ask for. This seems to be linked to the idea that the inner center is a balancing agent and sends the symbols or guides that people need to balance their life at any particular time. If a person enjoys and benefits from the guide experience, he or she can get other guides to meet other needs.

People meet guides through various means. Sometimes they come in dreams or visions. In this case they may be sought after or come unbidden. More commonly, especially in our culture, people encounter their guides in a reverie state during an imagery exercise designed for receiving a guide. In any event, a person can make a purposeful decision to get a guide, and exert great effort on that behalf. In tribal times ordeals were used during a vision quest whose goal was to get a guide. People would go to a remote place where they went without food, water, or shelter. In this arduous situation they would make an emotional entreaty for a guide and then wait patiently, for days if necessary, until a guide appeared in a vision. They might have to embark on a vision quest more than once. Scientists now believe that fasting, extremes of cold and heat, and listening to repeated rapid drumming help put people into reverie states in which they are more likely to have visionary experiences. In a real sense an illness can function in the same way. The suffering entailed when the body is not well motivates people to seek relief and puts them in an altered state of consciousness. Suffering makes people receptive to new ideas and motivates them to undertake changes.

Some people readily meet guides the first time they do a programmed exercise, while others encounter guides more easily during less directed exercises, such as drumming or gonging. When people meet guides easily, it's almost as if the guide relationship is natural to them, or they've been waiting for one. It is also possible that getting a guide is facilitated by prior imagery exercises or natural imaging abilities. For other people it takes several exercises over a period of time before they meet a guide. Some people don't meet a guide easily. A person needs to put effort into the experience but should accept whatever comes out of it. It's not necessarily better for a person to get a guide than not to, because much of the guide work can be done through reverie states without a guide. I also believe that people will get a guide when they're meant to and that for some individuals guides may not be the best way to work with inner material.

The guide experience is not without problems. Some people have difficulty seeing the whole of their guide; some people have difficulty separating the guide's voice from their own. Many people have such high expectations about meeting a guide that they develop a kind of performance anxiety during the exercise and become blocked. They want very much to meet a guide and become very frustrated when the exercise doesn't work. In these situations I advise people to take pressure off themselves and relax. Whatever images arise during the exercise, they should follow them, not extinguish them. In pursuing fleeting or vague images, they may find that the images come more quickly and become stronger. Occasionally people get guides that frighten them or that they do not like. This phenomenon is uncommon, and it can be dealt with. People have a choice: they can try working with the guide if they intuitively feel it is valuable, or they can let the guide go and search for another one. If people have difficulty seeing or hearing their guide, they should go into a deeper reverie state or repeat the exercise at another time.

I believe that information from a guide has to be validated, just like information from any other adviser. First people have to build up a relationship of trust with their guide. This happens naturally over a period of time as the advice given by the guide proves to be correct or useful. People should not follow a guide's advice if it doesn't make sense to them—any more than they would follow someone else's advice if it didn't make sense. This is especially important when dealing with illness or important life changes. Often incorrect information from a trusted guide is not really from the guide at all but is "ego static," that is, a result of confusing your own voice with that of the guide's. When people are anxious or upset, they tend to project their own voice onto that of their guide. Usually this is recognizable because the tone and style of the guide's response changes.

Most people find the guide experience helpful and intensely enjoyable. After a conversation with a guide, people often feel energized and at harmony with themselves and the world. Working with guides changes your reality. It encourages you to rely on inner rather than outer validation, and it profoundly ties you to the inner center. You look inward as well as out, which significantly changes your worldview and personality. Having a guide means you are never alone. You are always linked to something deeper, and you always have someone to talk to. Like Jung, I feel that it is crucial to bring the guide's information out into the world, to act on the suggestions of our guides, and to implement changes in order to balance our inner center.

The Discussion

In this chapter we'll deal with three techniques for meeting inner guides, but a fourth technique will be implicit in the information. All of the guided imagery exercises we've done up to this point will prepare you for the inner guide exercises. Suggestions in earlier exercises to change aspects of a room you visualize and to have an imaginary conversation with someone directly prepare you for these exercises. And the guardian figure that appears in the personal myth exercise is a direct forerunner of an inner figure.

The first technique I'll describe is a guided imagery exercise similar to the ones we've done in the previous chapters. It is based on the psychological approach that Carl Jung developed for contacting his unconscious or inner center. Jung called this technique *active imagination therapy*. In my exercises, I also incorporate relaxation techniques from behavioral medicine and guided imagery techniques from yoga. The first exercise is very directed, but I purposely have left many open ends so that people can go their own way. This type of programmed guided imagery seems to result in people meeting guides they can converse with easily. Guides that are met in this first type of exercise are often direct teachers and healers. Generally they are useful in dealing with daily problems and are close by and accessible. These generalizations don't always apply, but they are derived from my experience in teaching many people.

The second inner guide exercise has shamanic origins and is based on the work of Michael Harner, an anthropologist who has written and lectured widely about shamanism. This exercise uses drumming, an ancient technique that recently has been found to synchronize brain waves and make it easier for people to go into an altered state. It is also exciting. When you listen to drumming, ride the overtones, that is, pay attention to the echoes rather than the drumbeats themselves.

This exercise takes its technique from the shamanic practices of a number of cultures. Guides met in this exercise are often primitive, physical, and feeling-oriented. They are rich with energy and often seem very real. While doing this exercise, people often partially merge with their guide and identify with their guide for moments. Guides from this exercise are full of power that transfers directly into you. They can confer courage, strength, and confidence, as well as mental and physical energy.

The third inner guide exercise has spiritual roots. Guides met in this exercise tend to be ethereal, even holy. They deal with a higher level and often bring out feelings of joy. There is a tendency to merge or identify with these figures for moments during the exercise also. The guides feel distant, in that they are not superficially friendly, but generally they are filled with great love. Their personality characteristics are often indistinct, in that they are universal. This exercise uses gonging, which, like drumming, has a direct effect on brain waves and produces a deep, altered state. Gonging has been used for thousands of years in Buddhist monasteries. As in the drumming exercise, pay attention to the overtones.

The fourth, or implicit, exercise stems from a person's interest in guides and from simply reading the exercises. Basically, when people expose themselves to information about guides, it becomes more likely that they will meet a guide of their own outside of an exercise, either in a dream or in a vision. These visions can occur anytime, while a person is daydreaming, exercising, or praying—whenever the mind can be somewhat detached. These "visions" may not extinguish external reality, and they may come across as thoughts. Some people simply hear a voice in their mind that talks to them at crucial moments, like a conscience or witness.

I hope you enjoy the exercises. Don't put pressure on yourself to meet a guide immediately. Give yourself plenty of time. The experiences in the three exercises are very different. Some people may get three separate guides; some may see little during one or another of the exercises. The exercises in this chapter are both directed and undirected. The first exercise is a guided or directed one, whereas the second and third exercises are unguided. In the guided exercise you are led with suggestions; in the unguided exercises your mind is free to receive or create the entire vision. Some people find one type of exercise easier than the other. For example, one woman found that she always got stuck on certain phrases in directed exercises, but the unguided ones always brought forth rich imagery. Other people have difficulty seeing anything in unguided exercises but do very well in guided ones.

In workshops I advise people who have problems with directed imagery to create their own. If one detail is not to your liking, substitute another. And if you wish, create your own set of instructions completely. If you have problems with undirected imagery, my advice is to make it up, paint it, create it—exert some effort to see the images. I always tell people to treat unguided exercises like clouds in the sky. Look carefully at what's around you, and when it starts to remind you of something, go with that image, just as you would attempt to see the whole animal clearly if you thought you saw one in a cloud. Suddenly the animal pops into focus. I've also found it helps if you name the object when you see it. If something starts to look like a tiger and you say, "Ah, I've seen a tiger!" it will help the image come alive. If you don't see much in the inner world, give shape to the shadows. If you see a shadow that looks like a tail, follow it and see the rest of the animal. Don't worry about these exercises. They're just like daydreaming or making up a story. Try to accept what you see without judgment. It's often a surprise. Be open to whatever happens, and enjoy it.

The Exercises

Exercise 7—Meeting an Inner Guide through a Guided Imagery Approach.

Find a comfortable space where you will not be disturbed. Sit or lie down with your legs uncrossed, your arms at your sides or resting on your abdomen. Loosen any tight or constricting clothing. Close your eyes. Begin by inhaling slowly and deeply through your nostrils. Let the breath out through your nose slowly and completely. Continue breathing in this manner, allowing your abdomen to rise as you inhale and fall as you exhale. As you breathe allow yourself to relax.

Now count from three to one. Take a deep breath in, letting your abdomen rise, and as you breathe out say to yourself, "Three, three, three." See the number three each time you say it. On the next breath say and see the number two as you exhale. And finally, as you exhale again, say and see the number one. You are now at a deeper and more relaxed level of mind, a level at which positive and loving energy flows into you from the universe. Accept these "gift waves" with joy and let them flow into your body as you inhale. As you exhale let waves of love pass out of your body to everyone around you.

Now we will count backward from ten to one, deepening our relaxation as we inhale and exhale. Breathe in. Say to yourself, "Ten," and as you breathe out say to yourself, "More relaxed." Breathe in again to "Nine"; exhale to "Deeper and more relaxed." "Eight . . . more relaxed. Seven . . . even more relaxed. Six . . . more relaxed." As you continue counting backward, imagine that a sparkling dust sprinkles over you, and when it touches you, you become very relaxed. "Five . . . more relaxed. Four . . . deeper. Three . . . deeper. Two. One . . . very relaxed."

You are now at an even deeper and more relaxed level of mind, a level at which you can contact inner guides. Say to yourself, "I would like to meet a guide. I want to use my guide to help me with ——. I know that this guide will help to heal, to balance my life and the world around me." Now imagine that in front of you is an elevator. The doors open, and you walk in. You turn around and look at the number panel. There are buttons that go from one to ten. This is a special elevator: the numbers refer to levels below you, starting with one, which is one level deeper. Think to yourself which level your guide might be on, and push that button. Let the elevator descend slowly to that level and let the doors open.

Look around you. A path leads away from you. It may be day, or night, or twilight. Follow the path downward. It leads to an area of intense energy. You can feel the energy in your body as tingling, or lightness. You may be able to see the energy as a fast-moving, smoky light. Allow yourself to travel to the center of the area. Feel the light around you, flowing into your body. Drift and let the light recede behind you.

Now imagine that you can create a special place where you feel at home. It may be a room, it may be a house, it may be a place outdoors. It may be in the country or the city, on top of a building or by a waterfall. It may be made out of granite, concrete, glass, metal, or wood. Or it may be made of trees and rock. Let the shape, size, and appearance of the area come from your heart. This special place is yours alone. Give yourself time to create your space. Look around you. Notice the floor or ground, the walls or surroundings. If you wish, you can bring to this place certain special objects. You can make a comfortable place to sit or lie down. It can be a chair, a couch, or a soft mound of grass. You can make a working surface. It may be a desk, a platform, or a large, flat rock. You can put some objects on your working surface. Put a writing instrument and something to write on. Put a vessel full of liquid, a crystal, a wand, and anything else that you feel is necessary. The objects on the surface are tools you can use in any way you'd like. If you wish, you can imagine that there is a magic screen. It may be on a wall, or a window in nature. Finally, if you wish, you can create a special door. It should be at least six feet tall and two or three feet wide. This door can be in a wall, in its own area of the room, in a rock face, or standing by itself outdoors. It should be a sliding door that opens from bottom to top.

Now look around you and invite your guide to appear. If you have created a door, you can slowly allow the door to slide upward, and as the door rises you will see your guide for the first time. Glance toward the guide as it appears. Notice details of the guide's appearance—face, clothing, size, and shape. If at any point you have trouble with the image, have your guide appear again. It is not uncommon for the image of the guide to be unstable, and even for it to change from moment to moment. Trust what you see, and let your inner center elaborate on the image.

When you can get a sense of your guide, allow the guide to come toward you. Even if you can't "see" the guide, you can communicate with the inner voice. Thank the guide for coming, and tell the guide that you are very happy to see him or her. Tell the guide you would like to ask questions, and begin by asking what the guide's name is. Wait for a response. Anything that happens is fine; if the guide does not talk, that is all right. If the name is unclear, ask again, or simply continue the conversation. The voice you hear will sound like an inner voice responding in an inner conversation. Now ask the guide if you can speak about concerns that you have. Let the guide answer. Ask if the guide wants to say something to you, and wait for an answer. Remain in this space, talking to the guide, for as long as you wish. Ask the guide if you can talk together again. Wait for an answer. Thank the guide for coming and giving you help. Let the guide leave. If you have made a door, let the guide walk through the door, and let the door close. Rest in your special place as long as you wish.

When you wish to return to your everyday state, gently move your feet and count slowly from one to three. You will return to your everyday state feeling relaxed, comfortable, and full of energy. Your body will feel as if it is in a comfortable, healing space. Each time you do this exercise you will relax more deeply and more easily, and you will find it easier to meet and talk with your guide. The feelings of relaxation will deepen, and the whole exercise will become more and more pleasurable.

There are many alternatives in the psychological approach for meeting a guide. The most common technique is to do a guided imagery exercise, taking yourself to a meadow or mountaintop in a light fog. When you are there, allow a figure to emerge slowly from the fog and come toward you. You may see the whole figure at once, or you may first notice some part of the guide—the guide's face or feet. Another variation involves relaxing deeply and simply asking for a guide to speak to you. This variation relies on inner conversation before seeing the guide. It is a very good technique for people who have trouble getting a visual image of their guide. After people get a guide this way, they can go back and try to visualize the guide through the fog or behind the door. Any imagery exercise that involves meeting a figure or hearing an inner voice is fine. If you did not meet a guide in the exercise above, try one of these suggestions.

After I do this exercise, I invite people to share their experiences with me personally or with the group. However, I feel that for some people the guide experience should not be shared, at least initially. It is personal and private, and sharing it can lessen the energy. In any case, I am always amazed and awed by the responses that people volunteer. Ordinary people with no prior guided imagery experience relate visions of great beauty and mystery. Often these visions are as surprising to the people themselves as they are to me. One woman, who had been diagnosed with cancer of the cervix and was afraid to return to the doctor, met a shrunken, elderly Indian woman as her guide. Having had no interest in American Indian material, the woman was surprised and somewhat dismayed by her guide. She had expected someone more like herself. The guide told the woman that her femininity and wisdom did not depend upon her cervix. This concept was reinforced by the Indian woman's beauty and femininity even though she was no longer young. This experience helped strengthen the woman's resolve to continue treatment.

Some people have a hard time with this exercise and see little or nothing, or don't realize the power and importance of what they have seen. An engineer with a Catholic background but no interest in religion saw Jesus, much to his great shock and surprise. The man refused to speak to Jesus and repeatedly tried to send him away. Finally the figure disappeared, and the man asked for another guide. He then saw a small green blob that was soft and light. This creature he found he could speak to easily. A nurse who worked with cancer patients saw the feet of a guide, but as the door she created rose, the guide disappeared. The woman became so frustrated and angry that she burst into tears. She berated herself for failing and felt weak. I tried to reassure her that she could do the exercise in another way and then meet her guide. In the next exercise, an undirected one, the woman had a vision that she felt was very important to her. She saw Spider Woman, a classic healing figure in American Indian mythology. She was taken aback by this vision because she had loved and respected Spider Woman for years but never expected that she would be privileged to have this figure as a guide. Seeing Spider

Woman made her feel powerful and whole and strengthened her faith in her ability to be of help to patients. She remembered those times when she had been most effective in her work and had a feeling that with Spider Woman behind her, she could be even more powerful. A psychologist in a workshop said that this exercise taught him something very important. He said that throughout his life, he had had a voice that talked to him whenever he needed advice. The voice had been basic to his existence, but he had taken it for granted and had never related it to other people. The exercise made him realize that the voice was actually a guide and that he could help others to have a similar experience.

This guided imagery exercise takes us to unfamiliar places, and it requires skills that we are not used to. It is important, therefore, to repeat the exercise within the next several days in order to reinforce the experience. Each time you do the exercise, you'll get better and better at it, and your guide will become more and more real to you. If you don't do the guided imagery exercise again, the skill will disappear, and you will probably forget the guide. Native American lore holds that if you do not talk to your guide, the guide will eventually leave.

In workshops I usually share with the participants some of my guide experiences. My first spirit guide was Braxius. He would talk to me about books and help me write them. Sometimes his voice was so clear, I could write down what he said word for word. He also answered questions about book structure and editing. On *Healing with the Mind's Eye* his voice was clear. It often seemed to me the book was channeled. Each morning before I would write with Nancy, he would tell me what to write and I would transcribe his words as notes. One day while I was hiking in the Sierra Nevada he told me to change the book's structure. The information Braxius gives me is specific. He is a guide for books and relationships. When I would have a conflict with Nancy and feel hurt, he was one of the most powerful voices for forgiveness, peace, and harmony. He was basic in helping keep our marriage together during difficult times. He became my deepest teacher about books and relationships.

In the years since I wrote with Nancy, I have concentrated

more on spirit animal guides. Owls, bears, eagles, beavers, and hawks speak to me now. I ask them about healing, about prayer, about medicine wheels. Each guide has an individual knowledge. For me, bears are about healing; owls, seeing deeper into the darkness; eagles, seeing in the day; beavers, working on one step at a time; and hawks, clarity. I have written extensively about these guides in *The Path of the Feather* and *Shaman Wisdom, Shaman Healing.* The inner voices of the guides are fundamental to my life. I would go as far as to say that the guides are the most important thing in my life. The guidance and information that they share with me inform who I am and give me wisdom beyond my small, petty personality. They are a gateway to the infinite, a powerful doorway to the earth's healing voices. Guides help me make decisions, help me make choices, and still help me with books and relationships.

The guide space is also deeply connected to how this book was written, because the voice of this book is like that of an inner figure. The book was written in a different way than I have ever used before. In addition to doing library research and interviews, I *dreamed* much of this book. Each morning I would awake early, and while still half asleep I would dream and see images that I would write down immediately so that I would not lose them. In this way I would dream two pages of one-line notes. Looking at these pages later, I would create full sentences, which I would read to Nancy. Sometimes Nancy would write the sentences down exactly; sometimes she would ask questions and we would modify the material. Because much of the book was dreamed, the material in it felt as if it came from outside of me. To me the voice of the book was clear, direct, and powerful. All I had to do was relax and let it speak through me. So in a real sense I feel that the voice of the book is an individual separate from me, the voice of an old man who was a healer long ago.

Because much of the information came through me, it has a more universal energy and less of a single ego. I believe that books have lives of their own, and even voices of their own. When I'm writing, I try to quiet myself and hear the voice of the book. Writing in this way is almost like talking to an inner guide and then sharing the conversation with you, the reader. Many artists and writers have said that the creative process feels like this. Carl Jung, in his autobiography, observes that at his best, he felt as if he wasn't doing anything, that the process was happening by itself; he was not consciously creating the work, it was coming through him. He didn't know, and I don't know, where the information is coming from—from an unconscious part of my personality or even from outside myself. Whatever the answer, learning from this process involves quieting the voice of our ego, or personality, and listening to something deeper. In effect, the goal is to allow something more profound to emerge by itself. In this book, then, there are several voices: my voice introducing topics, leading discussions, describing experiences, telling stories, and offering reassurance; the old man's voice giving clear theories and ancient rituals; and Nancy's voice, loving and helping us both. You may be able to hear these voices separately, or they may all blend because they are one.

Exercise 8—Meeting an Inner Guide through a Shamanic Approach.

For a shamanic approach, it is useful to have a friend beat on a drum or shake a rattle. You can also play a tape recording of shamanic drumming. A few people can also do the drumming or rattling themselves. The drumming should be a strong, unvarying beat of 205 to 220 beats per minute, which is maintained for ten to twenty minutes. This energetic drumming is hard work. At the end, the drum should be beaten sharply four times in order to signal a return, then rapidly beaten for a half minute while the return journey is accomplished. Many people who are able to relax deeply can do the exercise without any accompanying sound.

Find a dark and quiet room where you will not be disturbed. Take off your shoes and lie on the floor. Loosen any tight or constricting clothing. Close your eyes or put one arm over your eyes. Begin to breathe deeply, allowing your abdomen to rise and fall. Allow yourself to relax. Now picture an opening or hole that leads downward. The hole can be an animal burrow, a cave, a hole in a tree, or an opening into the ground or the water. It can be a door with stairs or a magic hatch. Any opening that leads downward will do. Look at the hole until you can see details in and around it, and remember what the hole looks like.

Now look clearly at the hole, go down through the opening, and enter the tunnel. Let your body move downward, either by crawling, sliding, walking, or falling. Sometimes the incline is gentle, sometimes it is steep. The tunnel may curve or it may be straight. If you find an obstacle in the tunnel, go around it, go through it, or go back and go another way. Let yourself move through the tunnel.

When you get to the end of the tunnel, you will emerge outdoors. Look around you. Examine the landscape to become familiar with it and to get your bearings. Begin moving into the world you have come upon. Now look around this inner landscape for a guardian spirit or power animal. Don't struggle to find this figure; it will appear by itself. It may show itself as a living figure or as a representation. You may see many animals or figures in the landscape. You will recognize your guardian or power animal because it will feel right to you. Very likely it will also appear several times in different settings. Once you find your guardian or power animal, you can talk to it and travel with it. When you wish to return, or when the drumming signals you to return, go rapidly back upward through the tunnel and emerge from the hole where you started.

This exercise can be done with more or less direction than we have given here. You can simply listen to the drum and tell yourself that you will go downward and may see an animal, or you can work with a very directed exercise that describes in great detail the tunnel, the lower world, and the figures to seek or avoid. Individual people will respond best to more or less detailed instructions. If you don't see anything with just the drumming, you probably need more direction. Follow any shadow you see in the lower world and let it form a shape. When a shape starts to remind you of an animal, follow that thought and look at the rest of the animal.

This drumming exercise is exciting and wonderful for most people. Its world is full and feels different from anything most people have done. Because of the suggestions in the directions, many people meet animal guides. The animals range from friendly raccoons to fierce snow leopards. One woman met a huge black panther that terrified her as it approached. It came up to her and licked her neck and picked her up like a kitten. This nurturing action was so unexpected it made her cry. The next night, while walking back to her room, she saw a black cat leap out of the darkness. The cat actually jumped on her back and licked her neck. The next day she was amazed to discover that no one else could get near this cat. Another woman, a psychologist, met male and female lions as guides. She was so frightened of them that she would not approach them or talk to them, so she dismissed them. Later she met a small rabbit. The next day, while the group was making masks of their animal guides, this woman saw the lions appear out of the clay. The lions would not leave her, and at last she accepted them and felt that she could deal with their power. The animal guides take us back to a time when people saw the world as full of spirits.

Exercise 9—Meeting an Inner Guide through a Spiritual Approach.

For a spiritual approach, it is useful to have a friend beat on a gong. You can also play an audio tape of gonging. Gonging has a unique, all-encompassing, whirling sound in its aftertones that can sweep people upward. Gonging is a traditional tool used to enhance meditation in the Far East. It is very, very stimulating. This exercise can sometimes be done without the gonging if a person is deeply relaxed.

Find a comfortable space where you will not be disturbed. Sit or lie down with your legs uncrossed, your arms at your side or resting on your abdomen. Loosen any tight or constricting clothing. Close your eyes. Begin by inhaling slowly and deeply through your nostrils, allowing your abdomen to rise as you inhale and fall as you exhale. As you breathe allow yourself to relax.

Now imagine moving upward. Allow yourself to rise through the air. You may move in a spiral, ascend straight up, or fly through your own effort. Keep going higher. Allow yourself to go upward. Finally you will come to a place where you stop. Look around you. You may see a shimmering imaginary flat plane, clouds, a landscape, or even doors or paths floating in space. Move around in this new area. Look around. Figures may appear through the clouds, through a doorway, or simply out of the distance. Let the figures move toward you and greet them. Allow the figures to talk to you if they wish. Remain in this space as long as you want. When the gonging stops, descend gently back to the point where you started.

This exercise can also be done with more or less direction. You can simply listen to the gong and see what visions appear to you. Or, like Buddhists, you can listen to the gong and picture in detail specific deities and the celestial realms around them. As you've probably found, the experience of ascent is very different from the experience of descent in the previous exercise. People love doing this exercise because it feels peaceful and full of energy. The sound of the gonging is otherworldly and makes people hallucinate easily. The overtones of the gongs mysteriously move around the room like spirits. Because I suggest an ascent experience with gonging, the visions that arise tend to deal with space and the universe. At this point people often feel as if their consciousness is out of their body. A psychotherapist who worked with cancer patients said that during this exercise she clearly felt for the first time that she was out of her body. She felt as if she was up near the ceiling of the room and could see her body resting below. At this point she became anxious and immediately found herself back in her body. In my experience, I've found that whatever out-of-body feelings may represent, the experiences can be healing and meaningful to the individual.

Another person, during this exercise, saw himself picked up by a huge bird and carried upward to a mountaintop. There he became a baby bird and was put in a nest and fed. Another man with AIDS saw a vision of the universe breathing. He felt himself going out with the exhale as the universe was created, and coming back into the source as the universe was destroyed. He felt that this experience helped him understand the natural birth and death of all living things. This was deeply reassuring to him; it relieved tension and helped allay his fears. Somehow, simply seeing this vision of himself as connected to the creation of the world made him feel safer and cut through his sense of isolation.

This ends Part One, *Joy and Delight—Ah-h.* Relax . . . take some deep breaths. In this section we have done a great deal of work and progressed on our journey. We have made the inner world more accessible and have made guided imagery part of our lives. Trust the universe and see the sacred all around you. Feel your own power. Ground yourself solidly and return to the outer world relaxed and energized. Take a walk outdoors in nature. Feel the land heal you. See the glory around you and give love to the people in your life. You are now different. The world you see and create is different. Your new world is protected. In this tranquil place you can take a temporary but safe rest. This is the halfway point of our journey. In mythology, a rest at the halfway point is a special time. The hero has triumphed over some enemies, but he knows that the real work is yet to begin. He feels his new strength but knows how strenuous the road ahead will be. Although you have glimpsed unknown strengths in yourself, you know that much work remains. After this, the journey begins in earnest, so mentally prepare yourself to set out anew. Get your provisions and your helpers together. Have trust in the healing process. Let go. Let's go.

PART TWO

HEALING IN THE SACRED SPACE— AWE

5

THE LIGHT

This chapter brings us to a pivotal change in the book. We will progress from dealing with the reverie state, the state of being deeply relaxed, to working in the *sacred space,* the space in which profound healing takes place. In the first part of the book, we felt joy and delight as we "played" in the reverie state. We enjoyed following paths and crossing bridges; we rested and worked in our inner space. We shivered as we started our myth, and we were energized as we met our guide. We developed a tool to travel inward, and we built skills for deeper experiences.

In Part Two the work will begin in earnest. We will switch our focus from staying relaxed to healing illness, from learning new skills to using them. Emotionally this is a major shift. These spaces or processes are basically alike in that we go inside and change attitudes, but the energy necessary for healing a disease is much greater and requires more of us, especially if the illness is serious or life-threatening. With such illnesses, the tenor of our "play" changes. I use "play" here to refer to a drama in which we are a participant, a game in which we are a player, and the here-and-now way in which a child interacts with the world. In the case of serious illness, we feel an imperative to change; we feel a force urging us on. By "illness," I mean not only physical disease, but feelings of isolation and separation from a sense of oneness with the world, or confusion about our true path and who we are.

Healing, on the other hand, can be an ecstatic experience. The joy and love in healing are more intense than those involved in deeply relaxing or maintaining health. And it is also true that in most instances the suffering is more intense. For most people, initially it is the suffering and the possible concern with death that intensifies the process. Through this book, I hope that healing in the sacred space will serve to make joy and love more intense and to greatly lessen suffering. By "healing," I do not always mean curing an illness; at a deeper level, healing means improving a person's perception of life, restoring a person's sense of power and oneness and finding love. I view healing as a returning home, a coming back to a place we have lost. One of the things lost in illness is a sense of connection. Healing reconnects us to the inner center, reconnects us on a level that we may not have experienced before we became ill, and restores a oneness that has always been there but might not have been felt.

When we are ill, we want change. We want our body to be renewed. I believe that such renewal comes from the source of all life; the process of renewal is enhanced when we are able to feel oneness with, and tap the power of, the source. Healing empowers. Through love and transformation, healing brings us home. I use illness as a focus for several reasons. First, I am a physician and illness is a major concern for me. When I use guided imagery techniques, I use them most often with people who are ill, including those with life-threatening illnesses. I routinely see these techniques heal: I see people's lives changed, their attitudes and philosophies created anew, and their physical symptoms improved. The people I work with look more relaxed and younger, feel stronger, and are empowered. Because I work with sick people, this is my perspective on imagery work.

I also use guided imagery tools with people who are not ill. I work with health professionals who want to use guided imagery in their work and with people who want to solve problems in their life. Guided imagery works equally well with both groups, because the process is the same. A sick person is a well person with a physical illness. Both people are the same; both desire growth and a sense of well-being. Our path and goal are the same; only the focus is different.

In this part of the book "ah-h" changes to "awe." The feelings of joy and bliss deepen and change to an experience of mystery and power. We enter the realm of the *wholly other.* The sacred space in which healing occurs is a place of intense experience beyond language. It is a space in which we experience the fullness and majesty of something much greater than ourselves, a space in which we can see and feel that our own body is infinitesimal compared to the rest of creation. Most important, the sacred space feels different from the space of the everyday world. It is infused with energy and immediately produces a sense of interconnectedness and oneness. In the sacred space we lose our isolation and enter a different reality, in which, through our inner center, we are connected to all things.

The sacred space presents another paradox. In the sacred space all is different, yet all is the same. We are not in our world, yet we are still in our world. We are the same people we were, but we are also much more. We are affected by a power from inside us, yet it seems to come from outside us. To help understand this paradox, consider a stone. To most of us it does not seem to be alive. It seems separate, without feeling or connection. Now imagine a sacred stone, one that is imbued with power from a respected person. It may be a stone that Aborigines believe was part of a dreamtime myth, a stone from the mountain Moses climbed, or a stone containing a fossil of the first life on Earth. Suddenly the stone seems different; it's alive, is connected to us, and is capable of changing our feelings and emotions. It radiates power.

That is the difference between the two realities. One is empty and neutral, the other full and potent. A writer with multiple sclerosis told me, "When you live with a severe illness, reality is different. You are up against the demons for real. All is serious." This second half of the book works in the realm of the serious. The point of this section is to confront demons. You do not have to be physically ill to enter this realm; you just need serious intent. The intent can come from your own physical illness, from an illness in someone you're close to, from problems in your life, or from an intense desire for spiritual fulfillment. For all of us, the gift of this space is the real work that can be done here. Actual change is forced to take place. In workshops, some people come for relaxation and renewal, without expectations of profound inner change. Suddenly, unexpectedly, the imagery pushes them into a world where all is real. The seriousness of the work changes their reality. The world of imagery has areas of play and fantasy, but it also has areas of profound seriousness. Simply by experiencing the images with intention to heal, we enter this serious realm.

Healing takes place in a sacred space because our body and mind undergo transformation by themselves in this other mode of being. In the sacred space we feel comfort and lose panic; we feel support and lose our sense of isolation; we feel closer to the power that created the world, closer to the underlying cause of reality that created our bodies. We feel calm and quiet, yet full of energy. The sacred space supports our world. Its center is both a pillar and a doorway. The body recrystallizes and reforms as our world is re-created.

The sacred space is the organizing principle. It makes comprehensible the chaos that exists around us. The everyday world, by itself, often demonstrates little meaning or purpose. It is especially devoid of purpose in regard to profound questions such as why we are here, what death means, and what produces true happiness. The reason that the everyday world provides no answers to questions like these is that material objects are all of the same magnitude; they provide no reference point or center. All of the incoming sensory data they provide are more or less the same. In the sacred space, however, every object is different. Sacred space starts from a fixed point of reference, the world's center, from which all meaning is derived. Once we have a center to relate to, we can place ourselves and everything else in relation to it. Giving fundamental importance to one aspect of life, especially a deep symbolic or metaphoric aspect that underlies everyday reality, gives meaning to our world. Without it, it would be as if people walking down the street were to see only color, sound, and shape, and not see friends they love, a landscape they feel at home in, and tasks that have a purpose. A center gives meaning to the whole. A center is an attitude, a perception, a mental construct. From a center, we can heal. For each one of us, our inner center is the center of the world. Here, inner and outer are one.

To heal, we must cross into and through the sacred space and then go back into the world around us, transformed. The crucial point is crossing the threshold, and crossing from the everyday, or secular, into the sacred. Your spirit makes this journey, but your body follows. Entering the sacred space is very like entering the reverie state. It is a change, a crossover, an entrance. Like the reverie state, it is an inner space in which time and physical space expand. But whereas the reverie space is an empty, quiet space that you fill with your images, the sacred space is already full. It is pregnant; it is permeated with volition. Whereas the reverie state feels relaxing or stimulating according to the scenes you image, the sacred space feels urgent and full of energy. It contains a sense of terror in the face of majesty and power. There is a sense of tremendous alertness in the face of mystery and beauty. It has the excitement, deep emotion, and meaning of being with a lover. Above all, it is not ordinary. One is never alone in the sacred space; you are with a greater force. The sacred space itself is alive, and you feel its life as light and energy. Illness can be the motivation to get in touch with the sacred space, in touch with its power.

Sacred space is not homogeneous. It is not even continuous. It has breaks, holes, and crucial areas. With guided imagery, you enter sacred space through the hole in the center. Like the paradox of sacred space itself, the hole is both real and symbolic. The first step in the journey is to acknowledge that sacred space exists, and to know that the hole is there to enter. The next step is to make the decision to go through the hole. The third step is to search for and find the hole that leads into the center. The fourth step is to enter the hole. This entrance takes action or force initially, but then you simply fall in.

Traditional peoples enter sacred space through a hole that involves images of ascent or descent. Often the hole is near or surrounding a pillar, tree, or mountain. Such images were present in shamanic cultures and most major religions. One is never far from the hole; in fact, our world is always situated at the center. Religious people seek to live as near as possible to the center. Our inner center is the world center. Most myths of creation and territory involve the gods giving birth to the world from a center, navel, or sacred point. Later, the people seek to live, worship, and heal nearby. In Judaism and Christianity, the temple or cathedral copies the cosmic creation, re-creating the center where God created the earth and first spoke to man.

Once within the sacred space, the magic of transformation begins. Transformation involves an alchemic dance of mind and matter. A change of consciousness takes place as a result of developing new attitudes and allowing new images to emerge. Images make body, mind, and spirit resonate. The universal myth and our own myth are released; we ritually identify with the hero's adventure and are transformed. The new attitudes, myths, and images change us—physically, mentally, and spiritually. When our consciousness changes, our ignorance is dispelled and we see ourselves as whole, as part of the oneness. A crucial point is reached, and we can spontaneously heal. Like the creative process, transformation occurs only after preparation and work. This is the period of *trying* to heal. It is followed by the transformation, which takes place by itself, like the illumination of a creative process. This is the *allowing* part of the healing process. During this process, our power returns. In shamanic terms, our soul or spirit is returned to us. As we merge with the oneness around us, we feel the life force and become aware of our energy, love, and positivity. The new myth we create tells us that we do not have to concentrate on suffering; we can concentrate on the love all around us. As we are transformed, our fear, negativity, and sense of withdrawal all disappear and are replaced by joy, positivity, and a sense of connectedness.

Body and mind transform themselves through a process that is almost magical. Healers report that their patients suddenly seem better: their outlook on life changes and their physical symptoms improve. People who are ill say they suddenly feel better, that all is different. The shamanic view of the process was that the healer found the patient's spirit or soul and coaxed it home. The spirit is the source of the patient's power. The symptoms of spirit loss are depression, passivity, helplessness, and regression to childish coping responses. Spirit loss also involves a sense of emptiness, of separateness or isolation. The person with spirit loss feels as if the web or matrix that connects him or her to the world has been broken. The intense discomfort that ensues drives a person to seek healing. The healer, in returning the person's spirit, returns the person's energy. The person again feels positive, empowered, able to make life changes, and reconnected to the world. Once the spirit is returned, the person again feels his or her place in the matrix or web. The reconstruction of the break in the web is the magical step. Once that occurs, the body naturally renews itself.

A metaphor for this process is that the physical body creates itself daily around an invisible mental matrix. Each day cells in the body die and are replaced in an orderly, remarkably complex fashion. The body that we have now is not the body that we had years ago, in that it is made of new cells. But the pattern remains basically the same. You can recognize someone you haven't seen in years, even though the skin, muscle, and bone cells have changed. Remarkably, just as a person's face is continuously re-created in the same mold, people's bodies often re-create chronic illnesses. The invisible field or matrix on which the cells organize themselves has yet to be explained fully by science. In fact, researchers have not been able to explain the mechanism by which cells in an embryo form the many different tissues in the body. All they can say is that at predictable stages in development, undifferentiated systems start to turn into muscle, bone, and so on.

Throughout history, people have simply described the process as being controlled by forces greater than themselves, or as taking place by itself. I believe that the body is created around a matrix that can be influenced by the mind. I think that when people are able to transform the mental image of who they are, their body will tend to shape itself in that new image. The parallel in healing is that when the spirit is returned, when its symbols reach consciousness, the mind changes and sends a message to the body to create a new body that is appropriate to house the returning spirit. At that point new cells grow in and chronic illness may be healed. A physical example of this takes place in people with heart disease when plaque is dissolved and arteries open.

People feel the transformation as energy and light. From the earliest times, the change in consciousness brought about by entering the sacred space has been experienced as a spiritual light. This light dwells within, in our heart, and without, in the whole universe. The light symbolizes knowledge, understanding, and change, and helps open us to the world of the spirit. The light is an experience. It is felt as perfusing our body and coming from it. It perfuses the world and comes back into our body. It is a manifestation of the energy. The light acts as our guide. By concentrating on it, we are helped to stay transformed. As we stay with the light we heal. The light moves, circulates, travels. As we move in the light and the light moves within us, we heal. As we heal, the *delight* of the reverie state changes to the *light* of the sacred space.

We see the light with our inner eye. At first we glimpse the light as small. It appears as a smoky brightness inside or around one part of our body. Then with practice, the light intensifies and moves. The light is connected to the energies of healing. As we see the light, our attachments to our illness are released, and we're drawn closer to the place where we are all connected. The source of all the light is connected in the void. There is a parallel for this phenomenon in modern physics. Early in the twentieth century, scientists discovered that light behaved both as a particle and as a wave. It was also found that all the energy for the waves of light came from the same source, from the Big Bang, or beginning of the world. From these discoveries in physics comes a metaphor for inner light's effect on the body: the light seems to get between cells, like waves of radiation, and purify both the cells and the space between them.

Again, history can ground us. The concept of inner light is unusual enough in this culture that a description of its universality broadens our understanding. I include details in this description because they are similar to experiences of people I have worked with. The concept of light has always been important in tribal mythology. Light has also been described as a phenomenon experienced by meditators of all religions. The Eskimos have a mystical experience called *qaumaneq,* or *lighting,* in which a person suddenly feels a mysterious light in his body like a searchlight or fire. This light allows the person to see in the dark, literally as well as metaphorically. Australian Aborigines believe that they receive a supernatural light in their body in the form of rock crystals. In ancient Indian religions, the supreme force, *atmanbrahman,* is identified with a light in the heart. Ascetics who practice yoga report that they experience luminous visions such as the sun, fire, lightning, crystals, and the moon. The Hindu religious text, the Bhagavad-Gita, describes the great god Visnu as appearing like a light. In the Bhagavad-Gita, the Lord speaks to the warrior Arjuna and then Arjuna asks Visnu to reveal himself in his true form.

> The Lord: Of course, with the ordinary eye you cannot see me. I give you divine vision. Behold my absolute power! . . .
>
> Arjuna: You, wearer of crown, mace, and discus, you are a deluge of brilliant light all around. I see you, who can hardly be seen, with the splendor of radiant fires and suns, immeasurable. . . . Your power is infinite. Your arms reach infinitely far. Sun and moon are your eyes. This is how I see you.[1]

Buddha said that the sign of God is the light that rises. And in Buddhism, the Clear Light symbolizes ultimate reality and is believed to be seen by everyone at the moment of death. Tibetan myths relate how the earth was created from a void that emitted a blue light. And in Chinese Taoist meditation, people practice circulating an inner light. In Christianity, baptism is referred to as fire, the Holy Ghost is represented by a flame, and Christ is believed to have a body made of light. Finally, there have been many people, poets and artists in particular, who have spontaneously experienced a vision of light, followed by a change in their worldview and a healing. Whenever people experience the light, they are transformed by it. Their world is changed from a secular world to a sacred one. The world that individuals see depends on their culture, philosophy, and religious beliefs. But the common experience is of change and healing in the face of the light.

The last characteristic of sacred space is timelessness. Just as physical reality is altered in the sacred space, so is time. Like sacred space, sacred time is discontinuous, that is, it has breaks and holes. I believe that when people enter sacred time, they in fact enter timelessness. They return to the beginning of time when myths were created, and live continuously in that timeless moment. They enter a mythical time made present. Sacred time, or mythological time, is paradoxical. It is circular rather than linear and is therefore reversible. Every time people enter sacred space through a ritual, meditation, or exercise, they return to sacred time, and leave the historical present. Metaphorically, in the sacred space we can view ourselves as traveling faster than the speed of light. For people who are ill, timelessness is a great gift. It extends their life, giving them a glimpse of eternity. One year of sacred time, one month of sacred time, is priceless compared to one year or one month of profane time. When there is no time, there is nothing to fear. Nothing is missed, nothing is shortened. Death stops historical time but does not affect sacred time. Moreover, in the sacred space people have all the time they need to heal. They heal in the eternal moment. In sacred space, time is perceived as "a succession of eternities."

In this part of the book we will deal with entering the sacred space, and the ways of transformation. Chapter 6 will deal with healing visions. We will create healing visions to free our own healing adventure and will use guides to help us on our way. In Chapter 7 we will deal with the main tool we use for transformation, guided imagery. We will use the image of the light and images of our body's healing resources. Healing energy fuels the transformation. Finally, in the last chapter, we will talk about power. We will allow the power to deepen by dealing with guilt and thinking about the meaning of death. We will glimpse our own transformation and bring what we have learned out into the world in order to start making changes in our lives. I hope that this part of the book will make you feel calm, peaceful, and energized. I hope it returns power to you and helps bring back your soul. I hope it allows you to heal yourself and be healed by the energy of the universe.

The Discussion

In the exercises for this chapter, we will practice being in a sacred space and work on experiencing inner light. The emphasis in these exercises will be on feeling. Through our feelings we will begin to understand what sacred space and inner light are. Some of us have been experiencing sacred space in earlier exercises, but now we will purposefully seek to do it. Certainly the initiation and inner guide exercises take place in sacred space. But since we undertook them in a spirit of play, some people may not have been aware of the power of the imagery. An engineer I worked with was having vivid imagery experiences that he did not understand. He would see a playing field, and then a forest, and then a boat. He didn't realize that for imagery to be most useful, he could ask for images with a purpose. He could approach the exercise with the intent to solve a problem or heal. When he repeated the exercises in this manner, he found that he understood the images and they were useful to him.

In the next exercises we will define our intent as sacred. Intent is our goal, our purpose, our mythological reason to heal, grow, or answer questions. Intent serves as a guide, a direction finder for our imagery. The first exercise is distinctly feeling-oriented. It involves practice in creating, feeling, moving, and using inner light for healing within our own bodies. The exercise is similar to those used in religious and psychological healings throughout the ages. This healing rite is cleansing and deeply energizing. Finally, the first exercise will allow us to experience various forms of inner light. This exercise is magical and nonlinear, deeply relaxing and comforting. In workshops I work extensively with the imagery of light. I've found that if there is one image that makes people feel better immediately, it is light. The images are not as personal or exciting as a guide or power animal, but they seem deep and basic.

The second exercise will celebrate crossing into sacred space. It will allow us to change levels in order to enter sacred space and reconnect with the beginning of time. It will also enable us to reconnect with mythological stories about the beginning of healing. I have found this exercise to be profoundly moving. People often reexperience previous visions in a more profound way; they see their guides or power animals but have more meaningful experiences with them. In this exercise the visions deepen and grow. Often guides reveal new information, and guides that have not spoken begin to speak. In this exercise, let yourself drift. Let the visions be your own: let your own figures emerge and your own myths unfold. When the elder speaks, see your own elder and hear your own story.

The Exercises

Exercise 10—Experiencing Inner Light.

Find a comfortable space where you will not be disturbed. Sit or lie down with your legs uncrossed, your arms at your sides or resting on your abdomen. Loosen any tight or constricting clothing. Close your eyes. Begin by inhaling slowly and deeply through your nostrils. Let the breath out through your nose slowly and completely. Continue breathing in this manner, allowing your abdomen to rise as you inhale and fall as you exhale. As you breathe allow yourself to relax.

Deepen the relaxation by counting backward from ten to one. Take a deep breath in, and as you inhale mentally say to yourself, "Ten." Let your breath out, and as you exhale say, "More relaxed." Breathe in, "Nine"; breathe out, "More relaxed." "Eight . . . even more relaxed. Seven . . . deeper. Six . . . more relaxed. Five . . . more relaxed. Four . . . deeper and more relaxed. Three . . . more relaxed. Two . . . even more relaxed. One." You are now at a deeper and more relaxed level of mind, a level at which you can travel and experience light.

Now imagine that you are in the country, in a place that you love at sunset. It can be at the shore, in the mountains, or near your home. Imagine that you are sitting with your eyes closed and meditating. The lovely feeling of this time surrounds you and fills your body. You are facing the setting sun; it is gently shining on your forehead. Feel the brightness behind your eyes and the warmth on your skin. Let the light flow into your body and move from your head down to your feet. Imagine that you are hollow. Let the light fill you from the bottom to the top. Imagine that your skin is transparent. Let the light shine out of you and into you. Now imagine that the light gets brighter. Imagine that you weigh very little. Imagine that you are floating above the ground. As you inhale imagine that light of all colors enters your body through each pore. In the moments between inhalation and exhalation, it is marvelously peaceful, and the light gets brighter. As you exhale imagine that light of many colors comes out of your body through all your pores. Imagine that the light radiates out toward the ends of the universe. As you inhale, imagine the light comes to you from the farthest places in the universe. Feel yourself expanding. Now imagine that the edges of your body are becoming indistinct. Imagine that the light in your body merges with the light outside your body.

Now imagine that in the center of your body is a point of light. As you inhale, light comes from far in the universe toward the point of light. And as you exhale, it goes from the point of light to the furthest corners of the universe. Now imagine that the point of light moves toward any illness you have in your body. When it reaches the illness, the illness is burned and disappears. If you feel tingling, buzzing, or warmth in that area, concentrate on that feeling. Let the point of light rest where the illness was; let it get brighter and brighter as you inhale and exhale. Now let the point of light grow to the size of your whole body. Let it get brighter as you inhale and exhale. Let the point of light grow as large as a house. Let it get even brighter as you inhale and exhale. Let it grow to the size of the earth. Let it get brighter still as you inhale and exhale. Let it grow to the size of the universe. Let it grow even brighter as you inhale and exhale. Now let it shrink little by little, until it's the size of a tiny seed. Let it get brighter as you inhale and exhale. Let it grow again to the size of your body. Feel your body weightless and glowing. Feel it healing. Stay in this state as long as you wish.

When you wish to return to your everyday state, gently move your feet and count slowly from one to three. You will return to your everyday state relaxed, comfortable, and full of energy. Your body will feel as if it is in a comfortable, healing space. Each time you do this exercise you will relax more deeply and more easily. The feelings of relaxation will deepen, and the whole exercise will become more and more pleasurable.

People usually find this exercise deeply relaxing. They report feelings of tingling, lightness, and floating. Sometimes the exercise stimulates feelings of being out of the body. People who are ill also experience pain relief and an increase in strength. After the exercise these people often look noticeably younger and less worried. They wish to fill themselves with light in the outer world and often lie in the sun. One of the reasons this exercise is relaxing is that you do not have to work to picture anything; you simply experience the light.

Exercise 11—Feeling Sacred Space.

Find a comfortable space where you will not be disturbed. Sit or lie down with your legs uncrossed, your arms at your sides or resting on your abdomen. Loosen any tight or constricting clothing. Close your eyes. Begin by inhaling slowly and deeply through your nostrils. Let the breath out through your nose slowly and completely. Continue breathing in this manner, allowing your abdomen to rise as you inhale and fall as you exhale. As you breathe allow yourself to relax.

Imagine you are on a path in the country. It is spring, and it is warm. The path is made of smooth, pressed earth. Grass and trees grow to each side of it. It is dawn, just before sunrise, and it is not yet fully light. The altitude is about four thousand feet. It is a high plateau, surrounded by much higher mountains. The path leads gently downward. Imagine you are walking down the path. Feel the soft, cool earth on your bare feet. Occasionally the soft grass at the sides of the path will rub against your legs. There are other people walking on the path with you. You are walking to a traditional celebration of the new year. This is the first time that you will be at this ritual because you have just been initiated into the ways of your people. It is now your time to enter the sacred space.

You can see the person in front of you and hear the person behind you. Continue walking along the path. It will come to a narrow stream crossed by a sturdy wooden bridge. Walk across the bridge. Hear your footfalls on the bridge like the sound of a wooden drum. As you cross over the bridge, you will feel calmer and more relaxed. On the other side of the bridge the path enters a small glade of trees, and the light grows dimmer. The air becomes cooler and moister. Suddenly you come out of the trees, into a mountain meadow about two hundred feet in diameter. The meadow is covered with soft, short grass, surrounded by trees. In the distance, at the four corners of the meadow, you can see the snow-covered tops of four mountains. Directly overhead is a bright star, which slowly becomes dimmer as daylight increases. The people on the path in front of you and behind you walk along with you to the center of the meadow. There everyone sits in a small circle. In the center of the circle is a bare area of pressed dirt. In the center of this place is a dark area.

As you sit in the warm morning air, close your eyes. The rising dawn slowly brightens through your closed eyelids. You feel the ground under you. You begin to hear a voice. It is the voice of an elder. The elder tells you about the beginning of time. You listen to what the elder says. First the elder describes the "unformed," the time before the universe took shape. Listen as the elder describes the void. Now the elder talks about the first presence, the first thing in the void. Listen as the elder tells you about the first presence. Now the elder tells how the first presence turned into light and how the light spread outward. As you hear this the sun rises and suddenly fills the meadow with bright yellow light. You see the light through your eyelids and feel its new warmth on your face and body. The light flows inside your body, and you feel as if you are glowing. Your body feels empty, like a transparent tube. Its edges are made of a field of yellow light.

You feel something being put into one of your hands, and open your eyes. You look down and see that you have been given a carved stick. Each of the members of your group also has one. The sticks are about four feet long and about an inch thick. They are carved with beautiful patterns that you recognize. At the bottom of the stick are patterns that resemble things that you loved as a baby. Above these carvings are designs of things that held great meaning for you as a child. And above them are carvings of things that are now special to you as an adult.

Everyone stands and walks toward the area of bare earth in the center of the circle. With their sticks, people start to draw a spiral that goes from the outside of the circle to the center. You follow the person in front of you around the outside of the spiral, scraping the ground with your stick in the same track used by all the people ahead of you. The people in front of you slowly spiral in toward the center of the circle. As you go round the circle you look toward the mountains at the four corners of the meadow. Their tops blaze in the sun. You begin to come toward the center of the circle. When you near the center of the circle, your eyes close. You step into the center and begin to spin upward. Your stick is still in your hand.

You spiral up, and up, and up. Feel yourself rise higher and higher. Slowly you come to a stop at a different level. You walk into an area that is filled with light. You see clouds above you and a reflection below you. The other people from the circle are around you. On this level, all the people look as if they were made of light. Their tubelike sheaths glow with light. All of you start moving effortlessly toward a doorway that appears ahead out of the mist. The doorway has pillars on either side. In front of the pillars are carved animals. You float through the door with the rest of your people and drift toward a distant area of light. As you drift, you become more and more relaxed. The area of light gets closer.

As the area of light gets closer you can see that it is a horizontal circle of light, about twenty feet in diameter, whose center is darker and concave. This is the dreamtime navel of the earth, from which healing flows. Around the outside of the circle is a soft rim that has depressions that contour to your body. There is one for each member of your group. You lie in your seat. The whole edge of the circle radiates light. Slowly the circle starts to spin clockwise. You close your eyes. Feel any illness in your body being removed. Feel those spaces left empty being filled with healing light. All the illness turns to light, and the light rises and disappears. In its place a new, pure light arises.

At this point you open your eyes and point your stick upward toward a point above the center of the circle. A beam of light comes out of the end of your stick. It joins with the light coming from the ends of all the other sticks and meets in the bright source of light overhead. This light gets brighter and brighter. The beams of light merge and form a cone. The cone spreads out over all the people in the circle and fills them with light and energy that will protect them against illness. At last everyone stands and walks to the edge of the light. The group starts to spin and spirals downward. Finally the spiraling stops and you land.

You see that you are back in the circle in the meadow where you started. You see the people sitting around the circle. You see the sun overhead in the center of the circle. You feel its warmth on your head and body. You feel its light spreading through your body, filling it from the bottom up. You feel as if you glow with light. You look toward the center of the circle. The dark area and the spiral are gone. In their place is a pool of clear water, reflecting the sun.

When you wish to return to your everyday state, gently move your feet and count slowly from one to three. You will return to your everyday state relaxed, comfortable, and full of energy. Your body will feel as if it is in a comfortable, healing space. Each time you do this exercise you will relax more deeply and more easily. The feelings of relaxation will deepen, and the whole exercise will become more and more pleasurable.

At the end of this exercise people often do not want to return to the outer world. The exercise is filled with strange and unique feelings in a world that is timeless and spaceless. One woman, a psychologist, saw herself surrounded by shamans, one of whom she had seen in a previous exercise. Before the workshop she had not been particularly interested in shamans, and her first experience with them had surprised her. Increasingly she had been looking for something to make her work more alive but had not yet discovered anything. In this exercise the shamans danced around her and gave her a staff that made her powerful. They told her what to do to heal others. They told her that she could heal with her heart, that her feelings would be a help to her. She could feel the energy from the staff radiating from her wrist to her shoulder, and felt strong and clear. Up to this point she had been afraid of dealing with physical illnesses in her patients and had distrusted her feelings concerning healing. This vision of the shaman's staff helped her move forward.

Another woman, a graduate student, had seen a figure across a lake beckoning to her in the spirit guide exercise. In this exercise the same figure crossed the water, talked to her, and touched her. The figure told her that she had great inner strength and would succeed with the difficult thesis she was working on. She was amazed by the figure's power. She had been happy in the guide exercise when the figure had simply appeared but was delighted here when the figure talked to her and touched her. Her thesis had been challenging, and she had felt herself to be at an impasse. To continue with the work, she felt that she needed more support than she was receiving from her professor. The appearance of this inner guide reassured her greatly and gave her optimism and energy to move on.

6

THE VISION

I believe that visions heal. They heal by freeing energy from our inner world, energy that fills us with power. Visions can free our autonomic nervous system to lower blood pressure and make our heart rate regular, and free our immune system to fight infection or kill cancer cells. When we experience crucial images from the inner center, a connection is made between our inner center and our ego. When those images come to awareness, the inner and outer world are joined and brought into balance. This balance is echoed in our body, in our autonomic nervous system and in our immune system.

A physical metaphor for this process is crystallization. When a solution containing the proper ingredients is tapped or its temperature altered slightly, beautiful crystals suddenly begin to form and spread throughout the liquid. Likewise, when an image emerges into consciousness, the mind reframes itself, the body's energies are renewed, and blood flow and chemical balances are altered. The images cause body, mind, and spirit to resonate, and the body is made anew. When an image is freed, tremendous energy is released. Researchers have not yet identified this energy physically, but we can feel it as intense emotion, excitement, a sense of peace, a buzzing or tingling vibration, or warmth and lightness. When an inner image is freed, energy is felt moving in the body in a fluid, symmetrical pattern.

Increasingly I have been helping people work with visions. The first work that I did involved guided imagery with landscapes and spirit guides. Then for years I concentrated on patients picturing illnesses and healing forces. Now I have returned to visions as a healing tool and combine them with physiological imagery. I have always used visions in my own imagery. During talks with my guides I have visions of landscapes, trees, and mountains. When I am ill, I also picture my illness and healing forces. When I have arthritic pain caused by gout, I picture my joint linings, my white blood cells, and uric acid crystals. I also picture hawks, shamans, and mountains. I believe that both types of imagery are necessary: visions reconnect us to our source, and images of illness can help to focus our healing forces.

This chapter and the next go together as a pair. They are designed to give you practical skills in using guided imagery for healing. In them I will concentrate more on exercise than on theory. As I've said before guided imagery is experiential, and you learn most by doing it. These two chapters are concerned with two very different aspects of guided imagery. This chapter deals with basic symbolic or metaphoric visions. The next chapter deals with specific images of illness and healing. Here in this chapter I refer to the visions as basic imagery because the images are general and highly imaginary. These images deal with fundamental, archetypal memories. Thus they free energy in a deep and primal way. I believe that the energy freed by basic images can be a powerful force that balances and heals the whole body. The goal of this chapter is to free this energy and immediately increase a person's personal power. The return of personal power enables a person to mobilize his or her healing resources and undertake specific healing tasks. This chapter is designed to increase a person's confidence and strength in the broadest sense.

The next chapter has specific exercises for changing physiology in the part of the body that is ill. It is a focal process that concentrates energy on one area. Both chapters help people change their body physiology. The first chapter frees the energy of the whole body, the second concentrates energy on the illness. Basic and specific guided imagery exercises are interconnected. Over time basic imagery evokes specific imagery, and specific imagery leads to basic visions. Ultimately the two act together for healing.

Energy is the key to both chapters. This type of energy can be likened to the *life force,* the energy that keeps people going, growing, and healing. It is the energy of volition in our cells. This energy is the energy of the universe. It is the energy of the Big Bang; it is speechless and undefined, and it reflects the whole. A metaphor for increasing this energy is that energy is available throughout the universe and a vision can act as an *energy generator.* The generator gathers up energy, concentrates it, and increases its power. Visions are able to do this because they are closer to the primal source of energy. Visions act as an energy generator by moving us toward concentrated areas of energy. We can feel the energy flowing into our body, filling us up, and expanding us. Images of restricted or narrow areas such as caves, of open areas such as meadows or mountain tops, of archetypal figures, or of beams of light seem particularly able to concentrate energy. Focal images of cells and organs seem able to concentrate energy on one tiny area of the body.

Images seem to bring people into more direct contact with primal energy by feeding their soul. Each person has images or visions that are crucial and meaningful. The particular visions depend on the inheritance of the species and a person's life experiences. Visions are of two basic types, which are inseparably bound together. First, there are memory visions of meaningful events from our childhood or our past. Second, there are imagination images whose contents come from a place beyond experience or from a combination of experiences that are put together in a novel way. Psychologists have long debated whether imagination visions can come from genetic memory, as Jung defined archetypes, or even from outside a person. Those visions of importance that release energy can be significant memories or symbolic imagination images that are totally new. It is these crucial images that have the greatest power to heal. We all have the inborn ability to get in contact with these special images. To do this, we need only go into a reverie state and summon those images. This is not to say that the images come immediately or that they come without work. Some of them are tightly protected. We recognize these images when we feel the energy they release.

Visions heal in several ways. First, memory images heal by providing us with positive memories of our past. These images strengthen our self-esteem, enhance our feelings of self-efficacy, and help to shape a positive view of the future. Memory images can also heal by helping us deal with times when we were hurt. Crucial events in childhood often produce characteristic ways of relating to the world. This is particularly true for people who were either physically or emotionally abused as children. Often such situations can be so harmful that they produce physical or mental illness, even years later. Essentially these are learned or conditioned negative behavior patterns. When people glimpse the root cause of such patterns, they are often released from their negative powers. After releasing the image, a person can allow a new image to form that positively resolves the situation. For example, a businessman with high blood pressure, who had been constantly berated by his mother when he was a child, saw a vision of being yelled at and experienced the pain of that memory. When he saw the vision, he felt his body tense and contract, and felt weak. Then he pictured himself explaining his feelings to his mother and was able to see his mother behaving more positively toward him. He realized that his mother was who she was and that he was not responsible for her personality. He began to understand that he could not change her upbringing or her ways of mothering. However, he could begin to accept her and to get in touch with the part of her that loved him, rather than the part of her that berated him. When he saw the love that she felt for him, he was able to relax and feel his own power. These visions helped him release his anger and contributed to a decrease in his blood pressure. Imaging the problem or its cause, seeing the healing tools that we have, and seeing those tools solve the problem is a basic way that we can use imagery to heal. This three-stage process works for both life problems and physical illness. With a physical illness, a person could see the illness, see the body's healing tools, and see the healing tools removing the illness.

Another basic way that a vision heals is a one-step process. Simply glimpsing a crucial image and releasing its energy can be healing by itself. It is as if the person sees the solution without seeing the cause. An example of this was an older woman in a workshop who had arthritis and was very embarrassed at the way she looked when she walked. One day during a relaxation exercise whose goal was to relieve joint pain, she saw a vision of herself flying. The vision made her feel as if she had been set free. Her pain decreased, and she became less fearful of people making fun of her walking. This image produced great healing even though she did not completely come to terms with the root of her feelings. The woman simply felt more capable of taking on new challenges. Some visions are so basic and so beautiful that they are intrinsically healing. Such visions are archetypal and imaginary much more often than they are from memory. These visions are symbolic of underlying forces and powers that support the universe. For example, if a person sees a vision of a figure feeding children, it can be a symbol of the spirit of compassion. In ancient days a concept such as compassion was often personified as a spirit or guide, and people believed that seeing a vision of the particular symbol was tantamount to being visited or blessed by the spirit. Many people who are ill need a particular spirit to heal them. For some it might be courage; for others, compassion; and for still others, peace.

The third way in which images heal is an ongoing process. Experiencing a hero's adventure in which the hero surmounts a whole series of obstacles is an example of this last type of healing process. A mythological journey is also deeply symbolic and ties us to man's archetypal roots and memories. In an adventure, an individual identifies with the hero and becomes that person, taking on the hero's power. The goal of a mythological adventure is to surmount an obstacle and come out stronger because of it. This change and rebirth is particularly healing because, in a struggle, as in an illness, it is crucial to go all the way through and experience a new beginning. It is important to convert consciousness to action, to bring back to the outer world what has been learned in the inner world, to change lifestyle so as to create healing.

One way that people can get access to personal healing visions is through inner guides. Inner guides act as helpers, leading a person to visions and freeing images inside them. Guides reassure, take away fears, and put people in a state of mind that makes them open and positive enough to see visions. Almost by their very nature visions are elusive, so to access them people have to become calm, open, undistracted, and confident. The guide and the space in which the guide operates promote these conditions. I currently use three types of guides for visions: spirit guides, power animals, and celestial figures. Exercises for meeting these three types of guides were presented in Chapter 4. In this chapter we will discuss and give exercises for using guides specifically for healing.

For most people, the easiest type of guide to access for healing is the spirit guide. This is because spirit guides are the most human—they are the easiest to talk with, and they think in the most logical, human manner. I've found that there are different types of spirit guides that can be used for healing. As I've said, all guides have specific purposes, and not all guides are specifically interested in healing. There are two basic types of spirit guides that are interested in healing. The first is the *protective figure*, the guide who leads you on an adventure to see a healing vision. The second is a guide who is an inner doctor. In *The Well Body Book* (1972) I called this the *imaginary doctor.*

An inner doctor is like a real doctor in that he or she is often capable of diagnosing an illness and making suggestions for its treatment. Both the diagnosis and the treatment may or may not involve allopathic medicine and its techniques, drugs and surgery. Diagnoses can include images, metaphors, body sensations, or actual conditions. Suggested treatments can include advice about nutrition, exercise, and even drugs and surgery. In addition to advice, an imaginary doctor may perform treatments in the realm of inner space. They may "massage" parts of the body, go inside and "remove" areas of illness, or simply "wipe away" the image of the illness. Like other inner figures, the actions of the imaginary doctor are spontaneous and seem to come from the figure, not from a person's own ego. It is very important that people using an imaginary doctor listen to what the doctor is saying and not censor the material with their own thoughts. Some of the imaginary doctor's statements may be nonlogical or very surprising, and there is a tendency for people to disregard such statements. As I said in the chapter about guides, it is important to validate in the outer world suggestions that are made by the imaginary doctor in the inner world. But, of course, anything that seems incorrect or sounds unusual should be checked with supportive medical experts, just as you might seek a second opinion concerning drugs or surgery. Like a physician, an inner guide is not always correct, but over time people will establish a relationship of trust in the correctness of their guide's advice that is based on sound advice in the past. Suggestions that can't do any harm can be followed with less validation, even if it is difficult for people to see why the guide is making the suggestion.

The inner guide who is a protective figure can lead you on journeys in which you experience visions of healing energy. These guides have an uncanny ability to transform reality so that everything becomes alive and full of magic. These guides can also take you on journeys in the outer world that have a similar purpose. They can alter your vision so that the outer world becomes alive and magical. It is even more important not to censor the journeys taken with this type of guide, although it sometimes happens because the journeys tend to be less logical and less likely to obey the physical laws of time and space that make up our usual understanding of reality.

The second type of inner guide that helps people to heal is a *spirit* or *power animal*. As we said in the chapter on guides, animals seen in the inner world are different from ordinary animals in that they often can communicate and have knowledge and power. Power animals function on a more primitive level, involving bodily sensations and fleeting images. In working with a power animal for healing, people often merge with the animal in inner space and go on a journey with it. This allows people to make the journey with special protection, power, and strength. Often during power animal journeys people see shaman figures dressed as the power animal they identify with. In this case they may alternately merge with their power animal and with the shaman. Power animal visions break through the plane of reality. They do not obey the laws of time and space and often pop through holes and folds in space and time, much as the action does in dreams. It is very important to go with the flow of a power animal journey, because our sense of the everyday is very likely to extinguish the visions. In power animal journeys people often see fleeting shapes. If these can be identified and/or followed, they can bring forth powerful visions.

The third type of guide used in healing visions is the *celestial figure*. These figures exist on a different plane from the other figures. In terms of healing, they function almost as holy figures or gods. They lead you to beatific visions, touch you with healing energy, and bless you. Often they come spontaneously, unbidden, when people have profound religious experiences during prayer or meditation. To get help in healing from these figures, a person need only ask. These guides often use light for healing and put people in realms of energy that are so intense that they can be felt physically. The experience of these figures is like a healing force taking care of you. People who have experienced it describe an incredibly intense and powerful event.

Often when people are ill, their energy is not great enough to begin healing. They need help from a source outside themselves. Trusted friends, inner figures, and healers in the outer world provide this help. Both give people energy by reassuring them that they can get better. This concept alone frees people's own healing energy and gives them the confidence to begin the healing process. Both inner and outer healers give hope, and hope gives energy. People believe that healers know what's wrong, know how to cure illness, and have the skills and tools to do it. People trust that there is help and that they can be healed. This faith gives people back their power and, in shamanic terms, returns their soul. A successful visit with a healer is one in which a person is freed from fear, darkness, and worry. After contact is made with the healer, a person leaves with renewed energy and power. The contact is felt as energy and has effects that are both conscious and unconscious.

The Discussion

The exercises in this chapter are designed to promote visions for healing. The most important advice is simply to experience the exercises, to *do* them. Enjoy the exercises and let them happen to you. Your body knows how to heal itself. You don't have to do anything other than take your ego out of its way. To maximize your body's ability to heal, it is helpful to release your fears, worries, and doubts and to identify and become one with your vision. Healing energy will be freed and your healing will be enhanced without doing anything else.

Some of the exercises in this chapter are more directed than previous exercises. Although they are more specific, the directions are meant only as a model to help you create your own visions and conversations with your guides. When you do these exercises, use the directions as a framework for allowing your own personal thoughts and images to surface. The exercises will come out very differently for different individuals, and the answers and visions you receive will be stimulating and surprising. As I've mentioned before, do not put pressure on yourself to receive profound answers or dramatic visions every time you do the exercises. There are times when the experience will be dramatic, but often it will be very subtle, and that information can be just as important.

Before experiencing the guide exercises in this chapter, you should have first tried the exercises in the chapter on guides. Those exercises, which led you to meet a guide, had many open-ended directions. This chapter emphasizes using guides for healing, and it does not contain detailed instructions for meeting a guide. People may get the same spirit guides, power animals, and celestial figures that they met in Chapter 4, or they may find that their healing helper is a new figure. If you did not meet a guide, you can do the exercises anyway and still benefit greatly from them. The images are taken in at a level below consciousness and are healing to the spirit. The exercises in this chapter can also be used to help heal other people. Instead of picturing your body and an illness you have, picture your friend's body and the illness that he or she has.

The Exercises

Exercise 12—Using an Inner Figure or Spirit Guide for Healing.

Find a comfortable space where you will not be disturbed. Sit or lie down with your legs uncrossed, your arms at your sides or resting on your abdomen. Loosen any tight or constricting clothing. Close your eyes. Begin by inhaling slowly and deeply through your nostrils. Let the breath out through your nose slowly and completely. Continue breathing in this manner, allowing your abdomen to rise as you inhale and fall as you exhale. As you breathe allow yourself to relax.

Now count from three to one. Take a deep breath in, letting your abdomen rise, and as you breathe out, say to yourself, "Three, three, three." See the number three each time you say it. On the next breath, say and see the number two as you exhale. And finally, as you exhale again, say and see the number one. You are now at a deeper and more relaxed level of mind, a level at which positive and loving energy flows into you from the universe. Accept these "gift waves" with joy and let them flow into your body as you inhale. As you exhale let waves of love pass out of your body to everyone around you.

Now we will count backward from ten to one, deepening our relaxation as we inhale and exhale. Breathe in and say to yourself, "Ten." Breathe out and say to yourself, "More relaxed." Breathe in again and say, "Nine"; exhale to "Deeper and more relaxed." "Eight . . . more relaxed." "Seven . . . even more relaxed." "Six . . . more relaxed." As you continue counting backward, imagine that a sparkling dust sprinkles over you, and when it touches you, you become very relaxed. "Five . . . more relaxed. Four . . . deeper. Three . . . deeper. Two. One . . . very relaxed."

You are now at an even deeper and more relaxed level of mind, a level at which you can contact guides. Now say to yourself, "I would like to meet a guide for healing, a guide who will help my body become well. I know that this guide will help balance my life and the world around me." Now imagine that in front of you is an elevator. The door is open and you walk in. You turn around and look at the number panel. There are buttons that go from one to ten. This is a special elevator: the numbers refer to levels below you, starting with one, which is one level down. Picture the number of the level your healing guide will be on, and push that button. Let the elevator descend slowly to that level. When the doors open, you will be at the place where you will meet your healing guide. The doors may open to your special place, your inner workshop; to an office; to a place outdoors; or to somewhere else. When the doors open, you will see, hear, or feel the presence of your healing guide.

Let the doors open. Rest a minute. Step out of the elevator and begin to look around. See where you are. Look at the ground, or floor; look overhead. Look to each side of you. Ask your healing guide to come forth. Thank the guide for coming, and tell him or her that you're happy to be there. Ask the guide's name. Tell the guide that you have an illness or problem you want to work on. Ask if the guide will help you with this illness. Tell the guide that you will describe your illness; wait for a reply. To help you describe your illness, you can create a mental image of your body, either in the air or on a screen. Show the guide the areas of your body that you think are ill. If you have pain or other symptoms, describe them to the guide and point them out on the image of your body. See if you can view your illness clearly on the image of your body. You may see an actual organ or an area of darkness or of unusual color. Try to visualize the area of your illness as clearly as possible. See if you can visualize its size and shape and, if you wish, its consistency. Show and describe clearly the illness to your healing guide. Wait for the guide to respond. At this point some guides may want to work directly on or in your body. Talk about this with your guide. If you feel comfortable about it, invite your guide to do it. The guide will move around in the area of your illness in a circular, massaging fashion.

Ask if your guide knows why you are ill. Wait for a reply. Sometimes this is a difficult topic to deal with, so the answer may not be clear. Not all illnesses have known causes. You can ask this question several times if you wish. If your guide seems to know why you are ill but you have trouble understanding the answer, repeat the question and be very calm inside as you listen for the response. Answers to this question are often symbolic, metaphorical, or even spiritual; they need not be taken literally. Now ask your guide how your illness serves you in your life. Wait for an answer. Ask your guide if there is a way to fulfill this need without the illness. Allow time for an answer to come. Again, the answer may not be immediately obvious; all illnesses are not related to psychological needs.

Now ask your guide how you can heal this illness. Listen carefully to the reply. Some guides will give specific sets of instructions, at great length. Others will ask to work directly on your body. Ask your guide if there are food habits you should change or foods that would be good for you. Also ask if there is physical exercise that will be beneficial. Sometimes guides will lead you through physical exercises, explaining each body motion. Ask your guide if there are stress reduction or meditation techniques that will help you. Have the techniques described in detail. Ask if there are imagery exercises that would be beneficial, and if so, have the guide describe them in detail. Ask your guide what you should picture and what to do once you can visualize a particular image or change. Ask if there are any life changes you could make that would help heal your illness. These might be as simple as walking more slowly or simply not rushing all the time, or they might be as involved as radically altering your diet or changing jobs. Ask your guide if the medical therapy you're receiving is helping you to its optimum and if there are other therapies that you could do in conjunction with or instead of your present therapy. If your guide doesn't know of any, ask if you should look into it yourself. Ask if your doctor or healer is a good person for you to work with and how the relationship could be improved. If you haven't gone to a doctor for a problem that you are worried about, ask the guide if a medical visit would help you and/or ease your worries. Ask your guide to give you instructions or advice when you are in your every-day state of consciousness, not just when you are in the reverie state. This is especially valuable where diet and exercise are concerned.

Finally, ask if your guide heals directly, either through touch, by entering your body, or with "gift waves." If your guide heals in this manner, relax deeply and let your guide do this work now. Let the wonderful feelings of healing spread through your body. See illnesses shrink or disappear. Let feelings of comfort replace feelings of pain. Stay in this healing state as long as you wish.

When you wish to return to your everyday state, gently move your feet and count slowly from one to three. After you return you will be relaxed and full of energy. Your body will feel as if it is in a comfortable, healing space. Each time you do this exercise you will relax more deeply and more easily. The feelings of relaxation will deepen, and the whole exercise will become more and more pleasurable.

There are as many different responses to this exercise as there are people. Some people have guides that talk to them immediately, before they even ask questions. For some people the guide asks questions of them. Still others find that they must ask their guide questions one at a time. My healing guide is totally different from my other guides. She is a woman who greets me and then immediately goes into my body and moves around. I can feel a sensation in my body more than I can see or hear anything. She then will work on the area that is ill, and I will feel tingling and feelings of numbness. It feels a little like a gentle massage inside. She then leaves my body, and without asking any questions, she tells me things I must do to work on this illness. Her suggestions can vary from taking medicine to doing specific exercises. Sometimes when I'm exercising, she gives me specific instructions, like a physical therapist. A writer I worked with, who had arthritis, had a guide who told him to hike in the mountains, pick a specific plant, and wrap it around a joint that was bothering him. She then told him to walk in a special way. Several days later he found that his pain had diminished, and he was able to walk more easily.

Many people think that the most difficult part of working with an inner doctor is learning to trust the answers. People often ask how they can be sure if the advice they receive is correct. I have found that this is usually not as much of a problem as people anticipate. The guide's advice almost always seems intuitively correct to people. Because guides come from our inner center, they allow us to get in touch with a part of ourselves that is often thought of as intuition. So in one sense we are being reassured or getting information from a deeper part of ourselves. For these reasons, the information a person receives is generally not unusual; rather, it tends to reinforce or reassure people about therapies that they are already involved with or interested in. I have found that the most common use of guides in this respect is to help people make difficult choices. For example, a woman that I worked with who had breast cancer was having trouble deciding whether or not to undergo adjunctive chemotherapy. She had heard valid arguments both for and against chemotherapy in cases such as hers, and her physician wanted her to be part of the decision. Her guide told her that the therapy would be beneficial in her case, and she was able to feel better about the decision. Finally, as the information that a guide gives us proves to be correct, our trust in the guide grows. Often there is no one correct answer in a situation but several choices that from a medical point of view are equivalent, or several complementary therapies that are not harmful but that are not accepted by all physicians. Guides can help a person make choices that will be most in harmony with his or her inner self.

Exercise 13—Using Power Animals for Healing.

Find a dark, quiet room where you will not be disturbed. For this exercise it is useful to play a recording of shamanic drumming or have someone beat on a drum, as you did in Exercise 8. Take off your shoes and lie on the floor. Loosen any tight or constricting clothing. Close your eyes or put one arm over your eyes. Begin to breathe deeply, allowing your abdomen to rise and fall. Allow yourself to relax. Now picture the hole you saw earlier in the shamanic guide exercise, or any opening or hole that leads downward. The hole can be an animal burrow, a cave, a hole in a tree, or even an opening into water. It can be a door with stairs or a magic hatch. Any opening that leads downward will do. Clearly observe the hole until you can see details in and around it, and remember what the hole looks like.

Now look clearly at the hole, then go down through the opening and enter the tunnel. Let your body move downward, by either crawling, sliding, walking, or falling. Sometimes the incline is gentle; sometimes it is steep. The tunnel may be curved or it may be straight. If you find an obstacle in the tunnel, go around it, go through it, or go back and go another way. Let yourself move through the tunnel.

When you get to the end of the tunnel, you will emerge out of doors. Look around you. Examine the landscape to become familiar with it and to get your bearings. Begin moving into the world you have come upon. This land is called the lower world. Now search this inner landscape for your guardian spirit or power animal. Don't struggle to find this figure; it will appear by itself. It may be a figure that you have met before, or it may be an entirely new figure.

Greet your power animal and thank it for coming. Tell the power animal that you have an illness or a problem that you would like to work on, and ask the animal if it will help you with it. Watch the animal for its reply. The reply may come in the form of words, sounds, or body movements. If you wish, you may ask the power animal questions about your illness. You can ask why you are sick and what needs your illness may fulfill. If no answer comes, move on; not all illnesses have a simple cause or fulfill a need.

When you are finished talking, move with the animal. Let the animal lead, and follow alongside. As the animal picks up speed let yourself merge with the animal. Slide into the animal's body. Identify with the animal. Now move with the animal. Feel the movements in your body; experience being the animal. See with the animal's eyes; sniff with the animal's nose; hear with the animal's ears; feel the animal's muscles move. Allow yourself to move with the animal for a period of time. As you do this, allow the animal's strength and power to flow into your body. Concentrate on increasing the power in areas of your body that feel weak or sick. Let the animal's power and energy flow into those areas and make them bright.

As you continue to move with the animal, begin to look around you. Your sight is magical, and you can see great distances. You may see a figure of a shaman far away. Move toward that figure. The shaman is dressed in the costume of your power animal. As you get closer, you realize the shaman is dancing at a healing. Allow yourself to leave the animal's body and move into the body of the shaman. Feel the shaman's healing power. Let the power flow to areas in your body that feel weak or sick. Move back into the body of your power animal, and then back into the body of the shaman. Now move back into the body of the animal again. You may notice that the animal and the shaman are connected by a beam of light. This beam vibrates with healing energy. Touch the beam of light with your hand. Let the energy flow into your body and light you up. Let it concentrate in the area where you feel weak or ill.

Now move back into the body of your power animal. Move with the animal back to the tunnel or hole that you used to enter the lower world. Come out of your animal's body and stand at the opening. Feel the power of the lower world flowing into your body. Thank your animal and say good-bye. Watch the animal leave. When you are ready, enter the tunnel and return to the everyday world.

Currently, people are very attracted to the concept of power animals, which is somewhat surprising in light of how little background there is in our culture for this type of idea. The animals seen in this exercise feel extremely real to the people. For this reason, large animals, especially those in the cat family, can seem quite threatening and may take a while to get used to. In my experience the animals are not dangerous, but it often takes an act of trust for people to approach them. Personally, I do not separate the power animals met in this exercise from animals that people are drawn to in the outer world. In the personal introduction in Chapter 1 I asked you to pick an animal that you feel an association with. Most people, when asked to do this, say there is an animal they strongly favor. Often they have pictures or figures of the animal. Many people wear T-shirts or pins showing their favorite animal and will even visit the zoo to see the animal. When people associate themselves with an animal, they share the animal's power and spirit. A South American shaman I worked with had people picture an animal in parts of their body when they needed power. He would have people picture a lion in their heart for courage, a gazelle in their feet for speed, and an eagle in their eyes for clear vision. Such aphorisms as "strong as an ox" or "brave as a lion" indicate our culture's recognition of animal powers. Finally, many people report having strange or unusual experiences with the animal they are drawn to. A car dealer in one workshop saw a deer as his power animal. In the exercise, the deer simply stood next to him and sent him feelings of gentleness and softness. The next day, on a hike, a deer came right up to the man and stood near him for several minutes without moving. The man commented that he felt as if he were invisible to the deer, or that the deer saw him as a deer. American Indian shamans believe that when animals behave strangely in the outer world, they may be spirit or power animals. My books *The Path of the Feather* and *Shaman Wisdom, Shaman Healing*, discuss using spirit animals for healing in detail.

Exercise 14—Using Celestial Figures for Healing.

Find a comfortable space where you will not be disturbed. For this exercise it is useful to again play a recording of gonging or have a friend beat on a gong (see Exercise 8). Sit or lie down with your legs uncrossed, your arms at your sides or resting on your abdomen. Loosen any tight or constricting clothing. Close your eyes. Begin by inhaling slowly and deeply through your nostrils, allowing your abdomen to rise as you inhale and fall as you exhale. As you breathe allow yourself to relax.

Now imagine moving upward. In your mind allow yourself to rise through the air. You may move in a spiral, ascend straight up, or fly with your own effort. Keep going higher. Allow yourself to go upward. Finally you will come to a place where you stop. Look around you. Put one hand out to the side; feel another, larger hand take hold of yours. The hand belongs to a guardian figure. The hand feels like your parent's hand felt when you were a little child. Feel the love and energy in that hand. The hand slowly leads you across the plain. As you move, the love and energy in the hand increases. You are led toward an area of white light; the light forms a circle with an open center. The light looks like white flames in a ring. In the center of the circle is a large figure; the figure is shining with light. You move near the edge of the circle with your guardian. The figure looks into your eyes, and you feel incredible loving energy flowing into your eyes. The energy flows into your eyes and into your whole body. Your body feels light and peaceful. Let the energy flow to any areas that feel weak or sick. Let the areas become brighter. Let the energy purify you as it flows down your body. Let it wash down over weak or sick areas and wash any illness away.

Remain in this space as long as you wish. When you are ready to leave, the hand of your guardian will lead you back to the place where you entered the upper world. Rest there as long as you wish. When you are ready to go, thank your guardian. Then let yourself slowly descend. Feel yourself touch the earth again. Rest a moment more.

When you wish to return to your everyday state, gently move your feet and count slowly from one to three. You will return to your everyday state relaxed and full of energy. Your body will feel as if it is in a comfortable, healing space. Each time you do this exercise you will relax more deeply and more easily. The feelings of relaxation will become more profound, and the whole exercise will become more and more pleasurable.

. . .

This exercise promotes unusual experiences in some people. One man that I worked with was a businessman who had had complications after major surgery. In the recovery room he began to hemorrhage. The way the doctors were talking made him realize the situation was critical. Despite all that was going on around him, he suddenly felt himself drifting upward in his mind until he reached a place where he sensed a strong guardian presence. He felt that the guardian was a woman who radiated light, and he believed that as long as she stayed with him he would be completely safe. He felt filled with light and far above his physical body. During this time he felt no sensation of pain and felt that he was in no danger of dying as long as he stayed with this guardian figure. When he returned to his usual state of mind, the crisis was over. In reflecting on this powerful experience, he felt that he had done nothing to initiate it but that he had truly been in the presence of a guardian angel. For that period of time he had felt indescribable peace.

Exercise 15—Using Childhood Memories for Healing.

Find a comfortable space where you will not be disturbed. Sit or lie down with your legs uncrossed, your arms at your sides or resting on your abdomen. Loosen any tight or constricting clothing. Close your eyes. Begin by inhaling slowly and deeply through your nostrils. Let the breath out through your nose slowly and completely. Continue breathing in this manner, allowing your abdomen to rise as you inhale and fall as you exhale. As you breathe allow yourself to relax.

Now count from three to one. Take a deep breath in, letting your abdomen rise, and as you breathe out say to yourself, "Three, three, three." See the number three each time you say it. On the next breath say and see the number two as you exhale. And finally, as you exhale again, say and see the number one. You are now at a deeper and more relaxed level of mind, a level at which positive and loving energy flows into you from the universe. Accept these "gift waves" with joy and let them flow into your body as you inhale. As you exhale let waves of love pass out of your body to everyone around you.

Now we will count backward from ten to one, deepening our relaxation as we inhale and exhale. Breathe in. Say to yourself, "Ten," and as you breathe out say to yourself, "More relaxed." Breathe in again to nine; exhale to "Deeper and more relaxed." "Eight . . . more relaxed. Seven . . . even more relaxed. Six . . . more relaxed." As you continue counting backward, imagine that a sparkling dust sprinkles over you, and when it touches you, you become very relaxed. "Five . . . more relaxed. Four . . . deeper. Three . . . deeper. Two. One . . . very relaxed."

You are now at an even deeper and more relaxed level of mind, a level at which you can explore aspects of your childhood. Begin with the age you are now. Look at your body; you are wearing clothes that you usually wear. You are about to go on a journey back into your past, a journey to times when you were younger. The journey has a special purpose. You will visit scenes that have had an effect on who you are, that have had an effect on the problems and illnesses that you have as an adult. You will be familiar with some of the scenes you see, but you may see other scenes that you had forgotten all about. Some of your younger memories may be upsetting or painful. Do not worry; you will see and remember only incidents that you can deal with and learn from. You may wish to take a friend or helper with you on your journey back in time. It can be someone you already know and trust, or it may be a new person or an inner guide. Look around you now and wait for a helper to appear. Greet this guide and tell him or her that you are traveling back in time and would like support and guidance.

Now let yourself drift backward in time. Drift until you reach a time that was meaningful and important for the problem or illness you are working on. Stop at this point and look around you. Notice how old you are and what you are wearing. Feel your body. Look at your surroundings and notice who is there. Now allow the image of a scene from this time to come to mind. Let the situation form and the action take place. Notice how you react to things that are said to you or about you. Be especially aware of how your body feels and how you are holding your body. Be aware of areas of muscle tension or pain. At any point that you wish, you can stop the action. You can talk with your helper and even have the helper ask questions or comfort you if you need it. At any point if you need to, you can rest or return to your present age. When you are ready, let the scene unfold.

When you have reexperienced a scene, you can begin to work with it. Now ask your helper or think about other, more positive ways this scene might have unfolded. Rewrite the scene as you would have wanted it to be. This is magic space, so the outcome can change, what people say or do can change, and even people's personalities can change. Our memories of the past, which are colored by our own viewpoint, affect who we are. We have the choice to replace illness-producing memories with more positive images. This allows us to heal ourselves and to look at the world differently in the present.

Now let the rewritten scene unfold. See yourself and the other people as you would like to. Tell people what you might not have said in your memory, and have people say the things you would like them to have said. If you wish, your helper can give you or the other people suggestions. Allow yourself to spend time in the new scene and see things clearly.

When you wish to return to your everyday state, gently move your feet and count slowly from one to three. You will return to your everyday state relaxed, comfortable, and full of energy. Your body will feel as if it is in a comfortable, healing space. When you are in your everyday state you will remember from this experience only things that are helpful to you. Take time to think over the experience and see the ways in which past events have shaped the way in which you and your body react to situations in the present. Think of your rewritten script and how it can improve your life at present.

Exercise 16—A Hero's Journey for Healing.

Throughout recorded time, stories have been used to help people heal. Heroes' journeys, in particular, are healing because their structure parallels the experience of becoming ill and getting well. The three parts of the hero's journey—separation, initiation, and return—correspond to becoming ill, fighting a battle against an illness, and healing. The concept of transformation or change is crucial to both the hero's journey and healing. Joseph Campbell, in *The Hero with a Thousand Faces,* has said that heroes' journeys have the effect of unlocking or releasing the flow of life energies into the "body of the world." In fact, Campbell believed that health depends on the flow of energies of the unconscious from inner to outer worlds, and that the hero's journey is a metaphor for this process. In the journey the cosmic order is continued through the flow of power from the source. According to Campbell, heroes' journeys have several common characteristics. The hero usually encounters a protective figure or figures. He or she has to cross a threshold into a zone of magnified power. There the person is tested with ordeals or obstacles. If successful, the person comes back to his or her original world transformed, with new vision and life-transmuting power.

Each of us is able to use the hero's journey for healing in different ways. We can do imagery exercises in which we imagine ourselves to be the hero. We can create our own myth, in which we see our illness and healing as a hero's journey. Or we can write, read, or view films dealing with the hero's journey. Each of these methods allows us to identify with the hero and frees some of our healing energy to flow from inner to outer. Here is an example of the beginning of a hero's journey. I wrote it to experience for myself what creating such a journey in fiction would be like. In this story I imagined that I set forth and proceeded to the beginning of an adventure. I wanted to encounter helpers and enter a dark kingdom; I wanted to glimpse my effect on the enemy and begin to see my own path. The story stops before I undertook battles and tests, and does not deal with my return. I include this story fragment in order to help people begin making up their own hero's journeys for growth and healing.

Making Up Your Own Hero's Journey for Healing: An Example. The earth was cracking, and I clearly saw the jagged crack appearing, the rocks falling down into it, and the fire below. This wasn't like an earthquake or an ordinary natural disaster; it was something much more profound. The earth actually was cracking and, in fact, probably was breaking apart. In the midst of my terror was a place of quiet, and if I rested in that place, I could almost hear laughter.

I awoke. I had been having this dream for years. It would come once in a while and shatter my reality. I was a photographer who had left my job to attempt a project that was both financially risky and confusing to me. For reasons I wasn't completely clear about, I had decided to attempt to photograph "power spots" around the earth. I didn't know much about what power spots were or where they were located, but I believed that this project was of great importance. I planned first to photograph American Indian kivas in the Southwest, and then monasteries in the Himalayas. I had once heard that these two areas were interconnected on an axis that was like the earth's spinal cord, and that they helped regulate the energy of the earth.

I had rigged an old Land Rover as a camera truck and had driven to northern Arizona in search of the first area. One morning as I was eating breakfast next to my truck on a high mesa, my dog started barking. I saw two figures in the distance, walking toward me. An old man and an old woman approached. The old man walked up to the truck. I stared into the old man's eyes and felt a feeling of recognition. I had met Povaji several years before, when the old man was lecturing in San Francisco. Povaji was a tribal elder from a rebellious clan whose new beliefs allowed him to talk to Anglos. In his lecture Povaji had told the story of the Hopi prophecy, according to which the world would end if people of good heart didn't work immediately to prevent the earth's destruction. The old woman had been at the lecture too. She hadn't said much, but I had felt much wisdom and power from her.

The man sat down and this time told a different story. He

said that according to his clan, the world had first been like a sea of milk. A snake had slept on the sea and had dreamed the earth, the stars, and the sun. The snake was lonely, so he dreamed the Ant people. The Ant people were huge and powerful. They made the mountains, the forests, and the seas. Some of the Ant people, however, became homesick. They wanted to return to their father, the snake, and the milky sea. They believed that if they destroyed the world, they could go home. The snake did not want them to come home until they had finished their work, and he became angry. The rebellious Ant people became more determined than ever and decided to destroy the earth by cracking it apart. Povaji stopped. I told him about my dream and about how upset I would become whenever I had the dream. Povaji continued. He said that the snake saw the crack and quickly tried to fix it. The snake developed a magical elixir and a song, which if used correctly could heal the earth. Again Povaji stopped. I felt uncomfortable with the story. I didn't understand what it had to do with me or whether it was true or real. I changed the subject. I asked Povaji where a kiva was that I could photograph, and whether the old man believed that local kivas were power spots. Povaji laughed. The old woman looked at me and pointed down the track that I was on. She said, "You want a power spot? Go down this road; you'll see a power spot."

I drove down the narrow dirt track and wondered where the woman was sending me. From my maps I knew that there was no major ruin or village in this area. I'd heard stories that there was a very old ruin of the first villages, which had not been excavated and which lay somewhere in this area, but there were no published descriptions of it or instructions to find it. My dog started barking. The dog lifted his head toward the roof of the truck and howled and grunted. I looked around and couldn't figure out what the dog was barking at. I stuck my head out of the window and looked up, and saw a beautiful hawk circling about fifty feet over the truck. The hawk dove, narrowly missing the windshield of the truck, then circled back up again. I continued driving on the track. Every so often the track would fork and I wouldn't know which way to turn. I would stop a moment, see the hawk circling one way or another, and follow its flight. I drove in this manner for hours. I must have turned at twenty or thirty forks, moving deeper and deeper into unknown country.

Ahead I saw a gleam of light. As I got closer I realized it was the sun reflecting off a new car. It was parked in the middle of an open area, and there was a sleeping bag and cooking gear nearby. I saw a woman dressed in a backcountry outfit. She had a pair of binoculars, a camera, and a notebook. I stopped my car and approached her on foot. I asked her if she had found any ruins in the area. She answered with a German accent and a voice full of suspicion, "Why do you ask?"

Despite how suspicious she was, I instinctively trusted her and immediately told her that I was looking for a power spot and had been sent in this direction by an old Indian woman. She sat down on a rock and was silent. She said nothing for several minutes. The hawk circled very low over us and then drifted to the east and landed on an outcropping of rock. My dog jumped out of the truck and walked slowly toward the hawk. The dog sat down about ten feet from the hawk and howled several times. The woman suddenly told me that she had come here from far away, that a teacher of hers from the Himalayas had given her fairly precise instructions to come to this place but had not told her what to look for.

It was starting to get dark. The woman and I sat together and talked. The hawk and the dog had not moved for over an hour. The woman's name was Tanya. She had been a tour guide in Tibet for a large travel company and had studied for a short time with a Tibetan lama. She too found herself drawn to this axis of power spots and felt compelled to seek them out. As it became darker, the two of us began to notice a strange light between the dog and the hawk. We walked toward the animals. As we got closer we noticed the strange light was more intense. It was red and warm.

When we reached the animals we could see that the light came out of a hole in the earth. Looking more closely at the area, we could see that the hole was square and outlined in stones. It was not a natural formation. The hole was at the end of a long rise in the earth that led away from us. The rise looked like a ripple or fold in the earth. It looked as if something had pushed the earth up from below. Glancing at it quickly, we could not tell if it had stone underneath and was unexcavated or was a natural formation. The square hole with the strange light appeared to be in the middle of a raised round area about thirty feet in diameter. Tanya and I walked into the circle and stood next to the hole. We felt tingling energy in our feet and were aware of warm air coming from the hole. We looked upward and saw four bright stars off in the cardinal directions and one very bright star overhead. I noticed that if I squinted, I could almost feel lines leading from the stars to the square hole.

The hawk suddenly walked over to the hole and flew down into it. The dog followed, barking and yelping. Tanya and I looked at each other as if to say, "Why not?" and followed the animals down into the hole. We dropped about six feet. It was now completely dark. The red light had disappeared. As we became accustomed to the darkness we could see that the space we were in was huge. In fact, we couldn't even see walls in any direction. The ground was flat but bumpy; the roof looked like the floor. Suddenly the red light reappeared, coming from the direction that the fold in the earth had led toward. The dog and hawk were nowhere to be seen. We heard barking from the direction of the light.

We started walking toward the light. The floor began to lead downward. As we walked, the light became brighter. It appeared to come from a square opening ahead. As we neared the opening, we noticed the dog was sitting ahead of us. When we reached him, he quietly walked alongside us. The square opening was a doorway. It had stone pillars on each side that were carved. In front of each pillar was a huge sculpted rat. The eyes of the rats glowed and followed our movements. The dog growled. The hawk appeared and landed on Tanya's shoulder. It stared into her eyes with fire and intensity. Tanya and I walked up to the rats; the rats hissed. The fiery light came from inside the doorway.

Suddenly, without warning, the dog attacked one of the rats, and the hawk attacked the other. Tanya and I ran through the doorway. The animals followed. It all took place in a second. When we turned around, the doorway and the pillars were gone. We could no longer see the hole we had come down through. The roof was no longer visible. Above us was a dark, smoky haze. The ground was rough and covered with rocks. Ahead was a deep chasm filled with fire. We felt an onerous presence.

We sat down. We did not know where we were or what to do. Wordlessly we both began to meditate. The dog lay down and went to sleep, and the hawk perched on a large rock nearby. I saw the chasm with fire in my meditation. It looked the same whether my eyes were open or closed. When my eyes were almost closed, I saw a strange vision. I saw hundreds of small red creatures with long, insectlike legs and wet, glistening bodies. The creatures were working furiously at the edge of the chasm. They had huge jacks that spanned the chasm, and they appeared to be working on the jacks, trying to make them expand further. I realized that they were forcing the chasm apart, making the crack larger. As the crack got larger, the earth shook. I recognized my dream.

Looking around, I saw a tube leading downward into the earth. The tube was filled with red light and appeared to have no end. A whistling, humming sound came from the tube. The creatures appeared to be taking directions from something behind them. I walked toward the edge of the crevice. The creatures stopped their work.

During conferences people occasionally have a vision that is so deeply moving that it electrifies the whole group. Such a vision can have a profound, immediate effect on a person's illness. A man with AIDS who was very ill and quite depressed had a vision of himself climbing a mountain. He climbed upward for hours and hours, becoming weaker and weaker. Finally he entered a narrow canyon that had steep, dark walls. As he entered the canyon his energy returned. He walked forward and found a large flat rock that looked like a table. For reasons he did not understand, he lay down on the rock and closed his eyes. Suddenly a beam of sunlight came down from straight overhead, filled his body with light, and flowed into his heart. He rested there until the exercise was over. For the remainder of the workshop, he felt wonderful. He was full of energy and felt intensely alive. The vision had changed his mind. It had changed his attitude from depression and hopelessness to joy and enthusiasm. Prior to the vision he had cried easily and had been unable to undertake actions easily. After the vision he was able to think about new therapies or drugs for his condition, talk about his illness with friends, and make plans for the future. I believe that the vision may also have strengthened his immune system and helped fight the virus.

7

THE IMAGE

In this chapter we arrive at our destination: using guided imagery for healing. As with all journeys, we have begun to realize that the path itself is the goal, the process is actually the destination. Up to this point we have increasingly immersed ourselves in the inner world of imagery. Each chapter has brought us deeper into this rich world and given us more extensive practice in experiencing its varied states. We started by playing in the reverie state, then we were initiated into deeper levels as we met our guides, and for the last several chapters we have been working seriously with symbolic healing. In the previous chapter we immersed ourselves in healing visions and thus began our conscious, deliberate use of guided imagery for healing. In this chapter we continue the adventure by applying guided imagery to specific illnesses. By now our skills have increased dramatically, and our level of comfort and our ability to move in the inner world have grown accordingly. Many of us are now at home in the inner world and are able to work there. Its images feel real to us.

In this chapter we'll use what we have learned to make images real. When we perceive images as real in the inner world, our body responds to them as if they were real in the outer world. When we believe that a piece of rope on the ground is a snake, our heart rate increases, blood flow to our heart changes, and our white blood cells' ability to fight infection drops for a short time. When we perceive specific healing images as real, our immune system's ability to fight infection and destroy cancer cells increases and our heart rate and blood pressure drop. Somehow the image actually signals each cell. When people imagine that they move their arm, microscopic movements can be detected in the muscles of their arm. It is likewise possible that when a person pictures white blood cells eating cancer cells, some sort of message is sent to the white blood cells and they actually start moving immediately. The message probably is a neuro-peptide released by the brain and picked up by receptors on the surface of the white blood cells. In this way, images might act by sending the body a message to heal. I believe that beyond such physiological parameters, something more profound and magical occurs when we see healing images as real. Picturing a healing image in your mind's eye changes more than your physiology; it changes your world. The healing image changes your perception of yourself, of your environment, and even of time and space. It unites the inner and outer world, and in doing so it releases energy. You feel the energy immediately, experience it, and become empowered. The feelings of empowerment and control further enhance the immune system and stimulate the parasympathetic branch of the autonomic nervous system to enhance healing.

Although this chapter is our destination, in a sense we've been here all along. You recognize the information in the previous paragraph; it's been at the heart of every chapter throughout the book. Nevertheless, this chapter does represent a real change. Now we will learn to create, hold, and make use of specific images for healing. We refer to such images as white blood cells eating cancer cells as "specific images" because they evoke predictable physiological changes. An image of an ice cube in the palm of your hand will drop the temperature of your skin; an image of resting will lower your heart rate; and an image of neutrophils, a type of white blood cell, eating cancer cells changes the number of neutrophils in your blood. In the last two chapters, images of white light and celestial figures or power animals were designed to produce healing in more basic and general ways. Here we are aiming at specific conditions; we are concerned with action. Our goal is to promote healing and to make us feel powerful and self-reliant by dealing directly with the disease.

First I want to introduce some imagery vocabulary. This vocabulary will give us tools to make images more useful and powerful. Imagery researchers use two terms that are valuable for us: vividness and controllability. An image is *vivid* when it seems real. It doesn't look "real" like a Technicolor movie, because life is not like a movie. It feels real because we can identify with it. An image is real when you momentarily forget the outer world, when you become so involved in the image that it momentarily becomes your world. That is not to say that you forget about the outer world; you always know in one part of your mind that you are sitting in a room doing imagery exercises, and you could always return to the outer world if necessary. But when you are imaging, for those moments the image is real. For some people one sense is stronger at imaging and makes the image more real. The image can be seen more clearly, heard more clearly, or felt more clearly. Exercise 1 will give you a feeling as to whether one of your senses is stronger than another. Vividness of imagery definitely increases with practice and time. The more time you spend at imagery, the more vivid the images will appear. Ideally, people should spend at least fifteen minutes to half an hour, two or three times a day, practicing their imagery. Once people become skillful at imagery, they can also use it effectively in short amounts of time. Although the image is real in the inner world, it feels different from perceptions of the outer world. Inner images are less distinct and more dreamlike. Do you remember the story of the woman who believed she could not visualize until I asked her to imagine tracing the letter "A"? Her comment was that she was surprised that that was all there was to imagery, that it was so simple. Imagery seems simple to us because our brain has evolved over thousands of years to process images. The right side of the brain has become specialized to "think" in images. However, our educational system has not concentrated on imagery, and most of us have not learned to image purposefully or consciously. Although we are often unaware of it, we image all the time as we make plans, create, and daydream. Imagery is not something new; it's something we do all the time.

Controllability is another important term that researchers use in reference to imagery. Controllability refers to a person's ability to change an image at will. It depends somewhat on a person's natural abilities and practice and somewhat on the particular images involved. Certain types of images have a life of their own and are difficult to control. For example, hallucinations and dream images are difficult to direct, whereas memory and imagination images are much easier to control. Like vividness, controllability increases with practice. At first images may be difficult to control, especially those that are emotionally charged. If you find that controllability presents a problem for you, meditation (see Exercise 3) will be helpful.

I use two terms that I feel are helpful for people doing imagery exercises. *Programmed imagery* refers to an image that we choose to hold and keep in our mind's eye. For example, if we wish to see white blood cells eating cancer cells, we can create an image of a white blood cell and a cancer cell and meditate on that image. Programmed imagery is highly effective, highly specific, and tends to be both vivid and controllable. Tibetan lamas taught elaborate exercises involving the programmed imagery of deities, body parts, colors, and light.

Receptive imagery refers to images that come by themselves, like pictures appearing on a blank screen. They are not invented or created, they are invited. Often it seems as if they simply pop into existence, like thoughts coming into your mind when it is empty. I believe that healing images come from the inner center and are self-balancing. These images arise in response to being called forth. When a person asks for an image to arise, a receptive image forms spontaneously. When people ask themselves what their illness "looks" like, often they see an image of cells or of a dark area in their body. These are examples of receptive images.

In reality, healing images are a combination of receptive and programmed images. As we image we invite and allow images to arise, and we hold those images that we are attracted to. When we try to visualize white blood cells healing an illness and we see an image of a shark eating a cancer cell and deliberately hold that image in our mind, we are using both receptive and programmed imagery. The combination of the two types of imagery is essential because in order for images to have healing power, they must be personal and meaningful. An image that someone else gives you may be effective, but an image that comes from the inner center is more powerful. We can tell when images have intensity by the way they feel. When an image is full of power, we become completely involved in it, see it clearly, and feel its energy. The image becomes vivid and alive, and we experience intense emotion or feelings of buzzing, tingling, pins and needles, lightness, or heaviness. When the image is very vibrant, our hair might even stand on end. People who are sensitive to energy can put their hands on or near a person who is imaging and feel when an image is intense or meaningful (see Exercise 17).

This discussion brings up the relationship between images and healing energy. Some people see, hear, or feel images; others have difficulty doing this but are aware of a change in mental state or of buzzing, tingling feelings of energy. Still others cannot separate the two experiences and often see the images and sense the energy simultaneously. I think that people vary in their natural abilities to see images and feel energy, and these abilities change with practice. When working with patients, I try to determine whether or not a person naturally tends to see images or feel energy, and I have them start the exercises by concentrating on what they are best at. In choosing exercises for a person, it is also useful to concentrate on skills the person already has. If the person has done relaxation for natural childbirth, I start with relaxation. By this point in the book readers have done a wide range of imagery exercises and should have some idea of whether they are more likely to see images or feel energy. Some people are better at guided rather than unguided imagery, or vice versa. For some people guided instructions are very helpful, and they see little during unguided exercises such as gonging or drumming. Other people block or resist specific instructions but experience rich imagery when they are allowed to pursue their own images. It is useful to choose initially those exercises that make use of one's natural skills.

Imagery is not a static process; it is dynamic. People don't see one image that stays fixed, but rather see a succession of images that form a process. Healing imagery is not usually like a single photograph; it is generally more like a movie. The succession of images are receptive images that come from our inner center. The ones we choose to concentrate on and elaborate on demonstrate our ability to control images. These are programmed images. The process that we image represents the pathophysiology of healing. It is like a small play in which the hero becomes victorious over an enemy. The choice of hero and enemy and the process by which victory is won are up to the individual and vary tremendously.

Basically, healers using guided imagery characterize the characters and the plot of the play in two ways. The characters of the play are either biological or metaphorical: either they are cells and tissues or they are symbolic forms that represent these structures. The process by which victory is won may be either aggressive (warrior model) or nonaggressive. The hero may triumph by violently destroying the enemy or by convincing the enemy to leave peacefully.

There are several different approaches that are used to teach guided imagery for healing. Basically, they vary in their emphasis on biological and metaphorical imagery and their emphasis on aggressive and nonaggressive processes. These approaches depend on the personal experiences of the healer, and since there are no accepted, randomized studies as to which approach is most effective, the choice is up to the individual.

The most common approach is to start with biological images. People are encouraged to learn about their illness and the physiological mechanisms that underlie healing. They can do this by talking to their doctor or healer and having the person explain to them in detail how the body heals itself from that condition. They can have the doctor draw pictures or show them models. In addition, people can read about their illness in medical texts or self-help medical books (see the bibliography). Books should be chosen that have good physiological descriptions and are not depressing about the possibilities for healing. Medical information is no longer secret; most medical libraries are open and accessible and now even make computer searches available. The Internet has medical information and you can find articles on any condition. It is important to recognize that the prognosis for an illness that is given in medical texts is statistical and does not necessarily reflect the outcome for any one individual. Physiological descriptions of both the process that causes the illness and the process that heals it are extremely valuable as models for biological imagery. In an earlier book, *The Well Adult*, we gave detailed physiological models for common diseases. One of the main goals was to give patients and therapists information that would be beneficial for imagery. Knowledge of physiological processes is especially important for psychologists and psychotherapists who are involved in treating physical illness with imagery. People are encouraged to study test results that picture their condition, such as X rays, MRI and CT scans, and laboratory values.

Based on specific physiological knowledge of their illness, people are asked to picture several images: first, an image of their illness; second, an image of their body's healing forces; and third, images of their healing forces dealing with the illness. People are asked to see the images in as much detail as possible—the size, shape, texture, and color of the illness and of the healing forces. Then people are asked to visualize clearly the action of the healing forces. Some healers have their patients draw a picture of these three images. Drawing helps people clarify their own images and note specific details. For example, a woman with breast cancer visualized her cancer cells as little black dots. They were near her breast, and there were not very many of them. She saw her healing forces as white blood cells with a mouth shaped like the creatures from a computer game. The blood cells were large and numerous. Her healing forces involved these big white blood cells moving around energetically and gobbling up the black dots.

What the healer does next is based on these pictures or on people's description of their imagery. The goals are to make the people see or feel the images as vividly as possible and to make people's images of healing forces stronger than their images of the illness. This phase is a crucial one and may take hard work. People must strengthen and enliven the image of their healing forces and thus allow the images of their illness to be weakened. Healers who have worked over long periods with many different patients believe that only when patients' images of the healing forces are stronger than the images of the illness will optimum healing take place. Finally, people need to strengthen and clarify the process by which the healing forces triumph over the illness. This process has to be clear, understandable, and physiologically correct. By physiologically correct, I mean that the basic process must agree with what actually happens in the body. Thus if an illness is the result of a suppressed immune system (for example, AIDS or cancer), one has to picture the immune system working harder. But if the disease is caused by an overactive immune system (for example, rheumatoid arthritis), one has to picture the immune system slowing down. Patients have to understand the healing process well enough to describe it to other people and have them understand it. If the process is not understandable, healing will not take place as effectively. For example, I encouraged the woman with breast cancer to give her cancer cells a personality so that they could be more easily recognized by her body's defenses. She saw the cancer cells as rough-edged creatures dripping with juice. They had little faces with frightened expressions. I also encouraged her to find the personality of her white blood cells. She said they had sharp eyes and an acute nose that could smell the juice of the cancer cells. She made them look ferocious and gave them even more energy for the feeding process. She could then see them as powerful enough to eat the cancer cells in a feeding frenzy. Her imagery was physiologically correct, in that large white blood cells do engulf and destroy cancer cells, and even identify the cancer cells through the use of chemical messages.

At present there is a debate among people working with imagery about whether or not healing imagery must be aggressive in nature. Some therapists feel that if their patients are to get better from life-threatening illnesses such as cancer, the people must use an aggressive or warrior model. These healers believe that the body responds more powerfully to aggressive images than it does to passive or peaceful ones. In fact, science has shown us that our physiology is aggressive. White blood cells destroy or kill virus, bacteria, and cancer cells. They inject these organisms with chemicals that dissolve the membranes of the dangerous cells and literally blow them up. Other healers believe that each individual has personal metaphors that free the body's healing forces most effectively, and that for some people peaceful images are the only ones that work. A current metaphor that is often used is that of the warrior. The warrior must perform each action impeccably, that is, with total involvement and ultimate beauty, being immersed in the here and now and making the most of each moment of life. Everything is devoted to victory, yet paradoxically the process, the form, is more important than the outcome.

I learned the lesson of the warrior from a lawyer with AIDS. He had attended a workshop, held by Jeanne Achterberg Frank Lawlis, and myself, in which he learned basic imagery skills. Following the workshop, he decided he must become a warrior, fighting to save his life, and that all his actions must become impeccable. He must endeavor to do each act perfectly, with beauty, for its own sake. Initially he started imaging wolves eating the AIDS virus, and pictured protection around his white blood cells. He also pictured killer cells eating the cells in his Kaposi's sarcoma. He did this imagery for the joy of it, without worrying about its effects. One year later he attended another workshop, at which I was teaching with Jeanne and Frank. The Kaposi's sarcoma was completely gone—it looked as if it had been removed surgically. His physician had followed the sarcoma and, because it was shrinking, had delayed surgery on it. When the sarcoma disappeared completely, the doctor was amazed. The man's white T cell count was normal, and he had no antigen activity toward the AIDS virus. He had taken AZT, the standard treatment, at the time while he did imagery. He felt healthy and strong and had moved from the city to the country and dropped the law in order to become an artist. He even began to lecture to AIDS patients on imagery and the warrior model.

Any way people can free their healing energies is the right way. But I have found that the great majority of people do this best with an aggressive model. Often people with peaceful models are not actually strongly imaging getting better. For many people, the peaceful models are not strong enough or clear enough to optimize their healing forces. Sometimes with a peaceful model, the healing forces are not pictured as being stronger than the illness. I believe that the crucial distinction lies in the strength of the healing forces, whether or not they are aggressive. You can say a prayer to the enemy, you can even validate them as being part of nature, but it is necessary to get the destructive cells or organisms out of your body. So the first part of the work involves building up the strength of the images of the body's healing forces and the process by which they work. This varies with the particular illness. Life-threatening illnesses need very strong healing forces. People need to work on these images for fifteen to thirty minutes a day, two or three times a day, for a period of months.

Healers that work with imagery have found that after a period of time, which varies with the individual, a magical transformation occurs. For example, white blood cells turn into sharks or little men, and viruses turn into tiny fish or rocks. The biological images turn into symbolic or metaphoric images. Thus the image of a white blood cell eating a virus is transformed into a process in which a shark eats a little fish. When this transformation occurs, the images become invested with much more energy. Not only does the process gain power because the images are made personal, but I believe that the symbolic images act in a deeper level of the brain and are more basic to human experience. When symbolic images appear, they have much more life than the biological ones. They are more energetic, and the process is more interesting.

People become involved with symbolic images because symbols have both meaning and emotion. It is easier for people to get involved with, identify with, and concentrate on images of this kind. The symbolic images change—the sharks grow, change color, multiply, and become more sophisticated in their hunting abilities. In other words, the stories themselves evolve, like a living being. The woman with breast cancer eventually experienced a transformation in her imagery. The cancer cells first seen as dots became mice who were dirty, weak, and sick. The white blood cells turned into huge, vicious cats. The cats were in a club and would hunt together for the mice twice a day. The woman also visualized mousetraps in her blood vessels and saw her chemotherapy drugs as mouse poison. She became very attached to the cats and hated the mice. As this imagery shift occurred she enjoyed it so much that she looked forward to her exercises each day. She said it was like watching a cartoon. She said the process actually took place by itself and was full of energy.

The model of picturing an illness and its healing forces in imagery that is initially biological and then metaphorical is not always used in a rigid form or used by all healers. In reality, no two people are alike, and each person's imagery adventure becomes his or her own. I encourage patients to be aware of the model above but to feel free to allow their own imagery path to emerge. When you are ill, start by allowing a picture of your illness to come to you. I've found that some people feel energy first, while others directly receive a metaphorical image without a biological one preceding it. I believe that most people actually have a mixture of biological images, metaphorical images, and energy sensations that are inextricably intertwined. To unravel them and concentrate on only one aspect takes away from the image's personal meaning and power. Likewise, when a person pictures the body's healing forces, those forces can appear as a mixture of biological and metaphorical images and body sensations. Many people don't even separate the images of the illness from those of the healing forces; they see them both together, interacting from the beginning. For a healing imagery experience to be effective, people must become one with the imagery. The more fluid and flexible the imagery is, the more likely this is to happen. So the model presented before is useful because it makes people aware of the different aspects that are important in any healing vision, but the model does not have to be followed slavishly.

I've found that it is often useful for people to have an inner dialogue as they are picturing healing images. This dialogue can be with any of the guides we've discussed in previous chapters or with any other inner voices people have. The inner doctor figure can be especially useful for this. One way the process works is that as people picture their illness they hear an inner voice making suggestions or asking questions in the background. The voice may suggest that an image be made bigger or advise them to make the healing forces move faster. Used in this way, inner voices add another dimension to imagery healing by allowing the inner center to further check and refine the images.

Many people find that, to their great delight, the laws of logic and cause and effect do not apply in the usual sense to biological images in the inner world. Instead, such boundaries are replaced by a surprising and exhilarating creative form of magic. For example, as people picture white blood cells beginning to attack viruses, the white blood cells may suddenly enlarge and multiply instantaneously, or they may suddenly grow faces, talk to each other, and change in shape. This spontaneous behavior of the body's healing forces is much like the behavior of a guide in that it happens by itself without people having to do anything. The whole story forms and grows by itself; we do not have to create it.

Healers working with imagery also find it very useful for people to incorporate into their imagery whatever medical treatments are being used. For example, chemotherapeutic drugs can be imaged as powerful bullets or voracious molecules, and radiation can be imaged as magic killer rays. In the same way, people can image surgery as successfully removing the illness. As we've said, the woman with breast cancer saw her chemotherapy as a mouse poison. During her treatments she would picture the poison flowing into mouse holes and dripping into little red cans. In the days after her chemotherapy she would picture the mice eating poison from the cans and becoming weak and dying. When imagery is used in this way it potentiates the power of the treatment and causes the body to work in conjunction with the treatment rather than to work against it. It also helps to lower people's fears and anxieties, which has been proven to lessen negative side effects. It is easy to theorize on the way in which imagery does this. Studies have demonstrated how imagery changes blood flow and muscle tension. When muscles relax and blood vessels dilate, the ability of drugs to get to an area is enhanced. Also, muscle tension causes pain and can make other organs work less effectively. So when muscles are relaxed, pain is decreased and other side effects such as nausea and vomiting are lessened. Healers have also found that picturing lab values on imaginary scales can produce healing.

People can focus on an image of the results of a lab test and follow the numbers over several weeks of imaging. Many people have found surprising correlations with the changes in actual lab values.

The most common problems people have in using imagery are not being able to see or feel images strongly and not being able to make the healing forces more powerful than the illness. These problems can be due to many causes. The simplest is lack of imagery practice or choosing an imagery modality in which you are weak. The initial remedy is to practice more and to use those sensory modalities in which you are strongest, whether they be sight, sound, and/or feeling. Another cause of imaging difficulty is lack of motivation. This can be caused by a person's lack of understanding or belief in imagery, or by imagery not being natural to a person. Some people are not comfortable with imagery or with psychological interventions in general. These people often do better with nutritional or chemical treatments. People who do not understand how imagery can affect the immune system often do not put much energy into the work. Sometimes a teacher can make the experience easier and more effective.

Finally, imagery for healing is not separate from the rest of the healing process. One's attitudes, love of life, and reasons for living play a crucial role in healing and deeply affect one's experiences with healing imagery. People who consciously or unconsciously want to heal may have less trouble picturing healing images or strengthening images of their body's healing forces. If people haven't dealt with the secondary gains or psychological issues around their illness, their ego may prevent healing images from surfacing effectively. It can be helpful for people who experience difficulty with images to talk with a therapist or inner adviser to clarify the role of their illness and remove this obstacle from their healing path.

In using biological imagery, a common problem that can arise is confusion over what physiological process to concentrate on. This is especially common where the illness is very complex and involves the immune system. For example, patients with AIDS worry about whether to concentrate on helper T cells or suppressor cells as new reports emphasize the role of one particular cell to a greater or lesser degree. Lewis Thomas, the former head of Memorial Sloan-Kettering Cancer Center, has said that he's afraid to image because he's afraid of choosing the wrong cell. I believe that this problem is less critical than some people think. For one thing, most people's biological imagery is not that precise. For example, an AIDS patient can simply picture anything killing the virus, anything protecting the immune system, along with immune system cells regrowing. Moreover, biological imagery generally switches so rapidly to symbolic imagery that the inner center essentially bypasses this problem. This natural way of dealing with the problem gives us the key to its resolution. There are several things people can do if they are worried about inaccurate biological images. First, they can check the correctness of the images with their doctor. Then, if they are still worried, they can allow their images to switch to more general or metaphorical ones. Finally, in this situation, people can use what we call *final-state visualizations*. They can picture themselves as well and whole, the specific tissue or organ having been healed. In fact, they can simply picture healthy cells in the area of the illness.

If people find that while they are doing healing imagery they become confused or depressed or find themselves prey to extraneous thoughts, especially doubt or worry, there is much they can do. First, they can stop the particular visualization that has caused the problem and invite in a more general, more spiritual image. This is the time to use images of white light, love, help, gift waves, or peaceful scenes. People can do a love meditation (Exercise 3) or a white light meditation (Exercise 10). In fact, any exercises from this book or elsewhere that make a person feel wonderful can be used to return power. Generally, the healing images that cause the most negative feelings are the beginning biological images because they sometimes lead people to concentrate on their illness rather than on their healing forces. People in this situation can focus on living or healing rather than on being sick. Finally, I advise people to concentrate on specific images, not theoretical concepts or phrases. In my experience it is easier for a person with heart disease to picture slippery arteries that plaques do not adhere to than to picture the concept of eating better.

. . .

A type of imagery that generally increases people's sense of well-being is *transpersonal imagery*. Transpersonal imagery deals with imagery between people, that is, when one person holds an image of another person healing. This type of imagery is probably the oldest form of healing. Shamans went on inner journeys in which they pictured the sick people getting well or their spirit being returned. Religious groups have used prayer and healing circles in which people picture those who are sick as getting better, and send them healing energy. Laying on of hands involves people picturing healing energy flowing from their body into the body of the sick person. Many Native American tribes believe that the more people who are present at a healing, the more likely the sick person is to get better.

For people who are schooled in the scientific approach, the mechanism of transpersonal imagery cannot be explained. When a person pictures an image and that image causes the autonomic nervous system to decrease blood pressure or stimulate immune function, a physiological pathway is traceable. A thought held in the mind results from excitation of nerve cells, which connect to other nerve cells, which affect the functioning of organs throughout the body. Although this sounds simple, the process is incredibly complex and has taken years to document. When people picture images of someone else healing, there are no nerve cells connecting their body to the other person's. No simple mechanical model supplies an answer. If patients know that someone is imaging their healing, it could be theorized that they will create an image of healing in their own mind or simply feel support and love that cause them to change their attitude. But if patients do not realize that healing energy is being imaged around them, there is no scientific explanation for how the healing energy works.

People who have used transpersonal healing have long explained its mechanism with philosophical belief systems. They believe that at deeper levels we are not separate; we are all one. They believe that separateness is an illusion taught to people by their culture and that in actuality there is only the great oneness or interconnectedness. The inner world, or reverie state, is closer to this oneness than our everyday consciousness. In the reverie state people feel their interconnectedness and feel boundaries disappear. They feel space and time dissolve, and the body becomes more diffuse. In the reverie state it is almost a natural feeling that images affect groups or systems rather than single individuals. An image glimpsed in the reverie state seems to be larger than one individual. When groups of people get together, images seem to come to them more easily and have more power. This is probably the reason that throughout history people have joined together to heal. It is a matter of firsthand experience. In all probability, the healing power of the doctor-patient relationship itself stems from the dissolution of boundaries between the two people and an increased feeling of oneness. Increased energy and energy flow accompany the feeling of oneness that occurs in groups. People experience energy moving from one person to another. There is as yet no scientific explanation for this phenomenon, but group healing is so enjoyable and so natural that its use is increasing despite the current lack of scientific proof.

Two types of transpersonal healing are in wide use. In the first type, the classic shamanic model, a healer images a patient as being well. The healer pictures the illness, the area healed, the illness disappearing, and/or energy flowing into the patient. The healer can picture either biological or symbolic images of healing or simply the healed state. The healer always does this as part of a ritual that involves a series of steps and special surroundings, which might include meadows and feathers in the case of some Native American healers or an office setting for a Western healer. Native American healers may also use sucking, tobacco, and cornmeal as part of their ritual. The healing may involve touching the patient, or it may occur at a distance—from close-up to far away. Healing over a long distance is obviously the most puzzling phenomenon for scientists. Basically, scientific explanations for this lie in parapsychology research. Many of the theories involve the behavior of waves and particles, the very frontiers of modern physics. For example, Robert Jahn, the dean of engineering at Princeton, speculates that the healer and patient develop a resonance between their minds. He suggests the possibility that electrons can tunnel through barriers without passing through the space in between.

The second type of transpersonal healing that is widely used is the healing circle, in which a group of people sit in a circle and touch or send healing energy or love to someone who is either in the circle or at a distance. As in any imagery application, people can use biological, symbolic, or final-state imagery. People who have participated in healing circles have found that both patients and healers are profoundly affected by such circles. People can feel energy moving around the circle, and can feel intense energy when it is directed toward them. The effect of healing circles is almost magical. The quiet of the circle is deeply relaxing, but beyond this, an intensity of feeling develops. The people within the circle feel deeply interconnected. The person being healed feels as if both individuals and the world are giving to him or her, while the people who are sending healing energy feel at one with the person being healed and feel that they are giving. The aura of receiving and giving seems to tie both healers and patient to the world around them. They feel they are getting a gift from each other. The experience of a healing circle is so transformative that it changes the group that uses it. It takes people out of logical, left-brain theorizing and away from worry and self-preoccupation; it puts people into an open, experiential mode in which they are tied to other people. The experience of the healing circle goes beyond words; it is simply felt.

I hold healing circles whenever I work with groups of people. I have found that the circle increases a sick person's energy and makes the whole group feel better. One circle that I held was done for a man with AIDS, who suddenly felt tired and weak in the midst of a five-day workshop. The man lay down, and each person in the group put a hand on his body. Each person sent him healing energy, and he pictured the healing energy flowing into his body. The group spontaneously started humming and then softly singing a song that one woman began. Gradually the whole group began to feel better. At the end of the circle we all stood and surrounded the man. He felt that his energy had increased greatly, and for the rest of the workshop he was able to participate with enjoyment.

The mechanisms by which a healing circle works remain a mystery, but one is certainly linked to the psychological concept of support. When people are drawn out of themselves and their ties to others are strengthened, they become closer to the oneness that underlies the universe. Just as reaching out to others in daily support prevents illness, promotes healing, and extends life for cancer patients, so may reaching out in a healing circle. In fact, the experience of the circle is generally more intense because it involves focusing a number of people on the same purposeful action. A second, more controversial mechanism for a healing circle is moving healing energy. People have long believed that some sort of energy comes into the body from the universe; this energy can be healing and can flow out and heal other people. Healing circles have people visualize energy flowing into them and then into someone who is ill. Individuals who are ill visualize energy flowing into them from other people in the circle. The act of visualizing in this manner can have a profound effect on the physiology of people who are sick. No matter what this energy is, or even whether it exists, the imagery process promotes healing. There is something about imaging energy that is especially healing. This effect may occur because such imagery is almost always associated with immediate physical sensations that can be consciously manipulated—moved, intensified, and sent out to others.

The concept of healing energy is extremely basic and ancient. Healing energy was referred to as *chi* by the ancient Chinese, as *prana* or *kundalini* by the East Indians, and as *baraka* by the Sufis. All of these cultures believed that healing energy was real and could be felt and moved by a series of exercises experienced in a reverie state. They also believed that disharmonies or blockages in the body's energies were a basic factor in causing illness. Freeing the energy from such blockages is considered to be an essential part of healing.

The most fully developed theories about body energy have been elaborated by Tibetan Tantric Buddhists. They believe that the energy called kundalini "sleeps" at the base of the spine and that with meditation techniques it is able to be moved upward throughout the body. Tantric devotees see the body as both real and metaphorical at the same time. Their explanation of the physiological processes involved use both metaphors and descriptions of structures. They believe that the body is made up of vessels or tubes, called *nadi,* through which energy can travel. According to Tantric students, there are thousands, even hundreds of thousands, of these pathways. The main ones are the spinal cord and the passages to either side of it. Tantric Buddhists also believe that there are centers in which the energy lies in a dormant state. These centers are called the *cakras* (pronounced "chakras"). The cakras are portrayed as circles or *mandalas.* A mandala is used by Tibetan Buddhists as a meditational device for centering. The word means "circle" and is drawn usually as a complex design comprised of a circle enclosing a square divided into triangles. The mandala expresses primordial unity and all the cosmic manifestations that make up life. According to Hindu tradition, there are seven basic cakras, which are loosely linked to nerve plexi along the spinal cord. The first, or root, cakra is at the base of the spinal column. The second cakra is at the base of the genital organs; the third at the level of the navel; the fourth one in the region of the heart; the fifth, the throat; the sixth, between the eyebrows; and the seventh, at the top of the head. When kundalini energy is moved, it rises from the bottom to the top cakra through the nadi, or channels. When the energy moves, it arouses intense heat. Arousing energy in the first, or root, cakra was believed to heal illness.

Traditional uses of healing energy and recent research aside, healing energy is a useful concept for people who are ill. I have found that most people who use imagery for healing feel energy moving in their body when they image. Also, many people who find they cannot hold mental images have an easy time feeling healing energy. I've described the feeling of healing energy many times throughout this book. As I've said, the energy feels like intense emotion, peace, tingling, buzzing, pulsing, throbbing, pins and needles, lightness, heaviness, or warmth. People spontaneously feel the energy appear in their extremities or in areas that are ill. People also feel it move throughout their body and notice that it has difficulty moving in certain areas. With practice, people can develop ways to circumvent these blockages or obstacles. Moving healing energy is one of the most exciting areas in imagery healing. It gives people immediate feedback through bodily sensations, and it distracts them from concentrating on pain or discomfort. Much more research needs to be done in this area in order to elucidate what physiological processes are occurring when the energy moves, and to explain how healing energy can flow from one person to another. Even before this research comes out, we can all make use of the valuable results of healing energy, both in working on ourselves and in working with other people.

The Discussion

The exercises in this chapter will focus on using specific imagery for healing. I will encourage you to explore biological imagery, metaphorical imagery, and final-state imagery. You will also practice feeling healing energy and moving it throughout your body. I hope that by trying the various types of imagery, you will be able to determine which forms are most natural, easy, and vivid for you. Although all the exercises are enjoyable, they require work. Visualizing an illness can sometimes be disturbing or upsetting. Often it brings people face-to-face with their own fears and doubts. Fear and doubt tend to extinguish imagery or make it less vivid. This problem is best dealt with by relaxing more deeply and working with whatever type of imagery flows most readily for you. Most guided imagery researchers agree that the most effective imagery is your own, that is, those images that come from your inner center. So a great deal of the work is to wait and watch images appear. The richness and spontaneity of personal imagery is surprising and exhilarating. The images come to you by themselves, without your having to consciously invent them. I believe that one of the most important characteristics of healing images is that they are alive. When images are alive they seem organic: they grow, change form, and move. This life seems to imbue them with greater power.

Most people begin healing imagery by seeing representations of cells and tissues. As I've said, before doing this it is helpful to consult a book on medicine, physiology, or healing for an explanation of your illness and the physiological mechanisms involved in its healing. Often the more people know about their illness, the easier it is to see images of it. One reference that many imagery workers have found useful is adapted from Dr. Steven Locke, the author of *The Healer Within*. Locke divides illnesses into two types—those with lowered immune function and those with excess immune function. Diseases with lowered immune function include infections and cancer; those with increased immune function include allergies and autoimmune diseases. It is important that people who are imaging their immune system know whether to visualize it working harder or resting. Another source of images that people find useful are the Lennart Nilsson books, which have beautiful color photographs of body tissues and white blood cells eating viruses and bacteria, and destroying cancer cells (see also *National Geographic,* June 1986).

As I've said, imagery gets easier with practice. The goal of a person's imagery work is to allow the healing imagery to increase in vividness and strength and become more vivid and powerful than the disease imagery. Often it is helpful to draw pictures of the imagery that you see. If any imagery makes you feel worse, leave it and go on to other imagery. If any imagery that you use makes you feel particularly wonderful, use it often. Finally, the imagery exercises in this chapter can be used for working to heal others. You can picture the illness that the other person has and visualize it disappearing. After doing this, picture yourself healthy and vibrant to optimize your own energy.

When I work with people who are ill, I talk at great length with them about their images. I look at drawings they've made, and together we develop a strategy to strengthen their healing forces and clarify the healing process. For example, the woman with breast cancer who saw cats eating tiny mice talked to me about making the cat bigger, making more cats, giving the cats a leader, giving the mice an odor and the cats a strong sense of smell, giving the cats knives and forks, buttering the mice, and developing better mousetraps or poison dispensers. The important thing is to have the person find an image that is both vivid and compelling and then elaborate on it.

The Exercises

Exercise 17—Feeling Healing Energy in Your Body.

Find a comfortable place where you will not be disturbed. Sit or lie down with your legs uncrossed, your arms at your sides or resting on your abdomen. Loosen any tight or constricting clothing. Close your eyes. Begin by inhaling slowly and deeply through your nostrils. Let the breath out through your nose slowly and completely. Continue breathing in this manner, allowing your abdomen to rise as you inhale and fall as you exhale. As you breathe allow yourself to relax.

First let your feet relax. Allow feelings of relaxation to spread to your feet. Become aware of any tingling, buzzing, pins and needles, or lightness that you feel in this area. As you breathe in allow those feelings to spread upward. As you breathe out let the sensations deepen at whatever level they have reached. Breathe in. Let the relaxation spread further up your legs. Breathe out. Let the feelings deepen. Breathe in. Let the feelings of relaxation spread to your abdomen. Breathe out. Let the feelings deepen. Breathe in. Let the feelings of relaxation spread to your chest. Breathe out. Let the feelings deepen. Let the feelings spread to your arms and hands. Breathe out. Let the feelings deepen. Breathe in. Let the feelings spread to your neck and head. Breathe out. Let the feelings deepen.

Now choose an area where the sensations of tingling or pulsing feel the strongest. Imagine that those feelings are flowing out to your whole body from that area. Let the feelings flow upward to your head and downward to your toes. Now imagine that the feelings of energy flow from the base of your spine up the right side of your spine to your head, and then flow down the left side of your spine, returning to the base. Allow the energy to rise again as you inhale and descend as you exhale. Now imagine that your spine is hollow and that the outside of it is thin and filmy. As you inhale imagine that your spine fills with energy. And as you exhale imagine that the energy radiates out from your spine to every area in your body.

Now imagine that you're surrounded by energy. Picture the energy as surrounding you like a radiant field. As you breathe in imagine the energy enters every pore of your body as tiny light beams. Imagine the energy flows to your spine and concentrates at the base. Now let the energy flow from the base of your spine toward an area of your body that you feel needs attention. As you inhale let the energy move, and as you exhale let it deepen. If the energy cannot move freely at any point and seems to have encountered an obstacle, imagine the energy goes past: the energy may go through the obstacle, dissolve the obstacle, or form new channels around the obstacle. The energy can strengthen before going through the obstacle or even send wires through it. Either let the energy find its own way around the obstacle, or consciously help it.

When the energy reaches that area of your body that you think needs attention, let it rest there. Feel sensations of tingling and buzzing increase in that area. Let the area relax. If the area is painful, picture the opposite side that is without pain, and let feelings flow from it. Now imagine that when you breathe in, energy comes in through the top of your head. You may even feel a slight feeling of pressure on the top of your head. Let the energy flow down your body like a gentle rain. Let the energy pool in any area that needs attention. Let it caress and cleanse that area.

When you wish to return to your everyday state, gently move your feet and count slowly from one to three. You will return to your everyday state feeling relaxed and full of energy. Your body will feel as if it is in a comfortable, healing space. Each time you do this exercise you will relax more deeply and more easily. The feelings of relaxation will deepen, and the whole exercise will become more and more pleasurable.

. . .

Healing energy is a concept that needs and deserves scientific study. When people rub their hands together, then hold them about six inches apart, they feel sensations of tingling or buzzing. If they do this with another person, they can feel energy from the other person. This kind of energy has been the basis for therapeutic touch and laying-on-of-hands healing. Some people find the sensation of healing energy the most interesting part of a workshop. They may go on to take other courses such as laying on of hands or therapeutic touch, and incorporate healing energy as one of their most valuable tools.

If you find that you can feel tingling or pulsing easily, you may want to try to feel other people's images. To do this, sit next to a person who is doing guided imagery exercises. Put a hand near or on the person's body, then ask them to picture healing images one after another. Many people pick up the intensity of the images by feeling tingling in their own body. In this way they can tell which images are most powerful.

Exercise 18—Using Specific Images for Healing.

Find a comfortable space where you will not be disturbed. Sit or lie down with your legs uncrossed, your arms at your sides or resting on your abdomen. Loosen any tight or constricting clothing. Close your eyes. Begin by inhaling slowly and deeply through your nostrils. Let the breath out through your nose slowly and completely. Continue breathing in this manner, allowing your abdomen to rise as you inhale and fall as you exhale. As you breathe allow yourself to relax.

Now count from three to one. Take a deep breath in, letting your abdomen rise, and as you breathe out say to yourself, "Three, three, three." See the number three each time you say it. On the next breath say and see the number two as you exhale. And finally, as you exhale again, say and see the number one. You are now at a deeper and more relaxed level of mind, a level at which positive and loving energy flows into you from the universe. Accept these "gift waves" with joy and let them flow into your body as you inhale. As you exhale let waves of love pass out of your body to everyone around you.

Now we will count backward from ten to one, deepening our relaxation as we inhale and exhale. Breathe in. Say to yourself, "Ten," and as you breathe out say to yourself, "More relaxed." Breathe in again to nine; exhale to "Deeper and more relaxed." "Eight . . . more relaxed. Seven . . . even more relaxed. Six . . . more relaxed." As you continue counting backward, imagine that a sparkling dust sprinkles over you, and when it touches you, you become very relaxed. "Five . . . more relaxed. Four . . . deeper. Three . . . deeper. Two. One . . . very relaxed."

Now rest with your eyes closed. Picture your body in front of you as if you are an observer looking at yourself from several feet away. Start by scanning your whole body. Let your eyes move from your head to your feet over and over again. Notice how incredibly complex and beautiful your body is. Feel its health and power. Now let your concentration move to an area that might have an illness or problem. Look around this area. The area may seem enlarged, as if you, the observer, were small. Look at the anatomy of the area in detail. Look at the color, texture, and shape of the tissues around you. Move around, looking at structures from different angles and vantage points. Allow yourself to move around the area and see how far it extends. Now concentrate on any other areas that don't seem healthy to you. Look at the details in this area. See the illness as clearly as possible: look at its size, shape, texture, and color. See if you can see individual cells in the area. As you look around, your guide may point things out to you or comment on your illness.

Now concentrate on how your body can heal this problem. Notice those tissues that create new tissue, fight infection, and eat cells that are old, injured, or unhealthy. Concentrate on your body's healing resources and watch how they work. Notice how they repair and heal tissues. Look at them in detail. Notice their size, color, shape, and number. Feel their strength and energy, and watch that strength and energy increase. See more healing forces come from other areas of the body. If you are taking any medicine for illness, imagine that the medicine comes to help your body's healing defenses. See the medicine coming to the area and watch it begin to work. See it kill microorganisms or unhealthy cells or relax cells in the area.

Concentrate on how your illness is healing. See new tissue forming in areas of injury. See microorganisms taken away and unhealthy cells removed. Allow this process to take place. It may take place slowly or rapidly. You may wish to repeat the process over and over, or let it work at its own speed. Now see the area completely healed. Look at the color, texture, and shape of the healthy tissue. Feel its strength and beauty. If the area appears abnormal or ill again, let the healing forces of your body work and make it right.

Let the healing process continue to work. You may notice that areas transform themselves from ill to healed and back. Let this go on and on. If the area stays ill, let a new type of healing mechanism work. If no new healing images appear spontaneously, ask your guide for help. When you can see the area as healed, feel the energy of the healed area. Let this energy expand and fill your whole body.

Now look at the illness or problem area from a different viewpoint. Let the tissues and healing forces become symbolic. Allow the structures to form anew; let them become objects, figures, animals, or places. This may happen immediately, or it may not occur until you have done the exercise a number of times. White blood cells may become strange creatures with giant mouths, blood vessel walls may become caverns, and viruses may become black dots. Let the image of the illness transform itself. Let the image of the healing forces also be transformed. Watch the healing forces deal with the illness. Let the healing forces become stronger, more numerous, and more powerful. Talk to them and congratulate them on the work they have done. If you have a guide, ask for suggestions on how to help the healing forces in your body. Let the healing forces become more and more powerful. You may notice that your imagery changes over time, that the figures alter in size or shape, or even turn into other things. Certain images may appear for short times and then be replaced by others. If any of the images feel particularly strong to you, repeat those images over and over again in your mind.

When you wish to return to your everyday state, gently move your feet and count slowly from one to three. You will return to your everyday state feeling relaxed and full of energy. Your body will feel as if it is in a comfortable, healing space. Each time you do this exercise you will relax more deeply and more easily. The feelings of relaxation will deepen, and the whole exercise will become more and more pleasurable.

This is the basic guided imagery exercise in the book that deals with specific illnesses. The material it contains is fundamental to imagery healing. You can take the material in this exercise and start to heal yourself immediately. A woman with a rare lymphoma read my guided imagery book, *Seeing with the Mind's Eye*, and Jeanne Achterberg's book *Imagery and Healing*, and decided to work with guided imagery. Her doctor had told her that, at that time, there was no treatment for the type of lymphoma that she had. She began by imaging white blood cells eating lymphoma cells. The imagery grew and expanded. She enjoyed the process and felt better and better. Now, years later, she is well.

This exercise can be done in many different ways. As we have said, some basic physiological research into your own illnesses and creating your own drawings is very useful. There is no question that the images that are your own are the most powerful. The images that are associated with the strongest healing energy seem to be the most effective. A woman with asthma pictured her trachea as a transparent tube. This image electrified her; it was so vivid that she momentarily became frightened. She then imagined that the tube widened. When she did this, her breathing immediately became easier, and she relaxed. She was very surprised by the power this image had over her long-standing asthma condition.

After you have done this exercise and made drawings, share the results with a friend or simply go over them in your own mind. Explain the healing process and see if it makes sense; criticize it as an observer. Ask yourself how you might make the image clearer, stronger, and/or more powerful. Ask what you can do to increase the power of the healing forces. For example, a woman who was infected with the Epstein-Barr virus drew a picture of round white blood cells eating little dots that represented the virus. In analyzing her drawing, she realized that if the dots were made clearer and more recognizable and the white blood cells were taught to hunt them out, the process would be more effective. So she colored the dots red, gave them hair, and made a school in which her white blood cells would be taught to recognize these hairy red dots.

Exercise 19—A Healing Circle.

Find a comfortable space where you will not be disturbed. Sit or lie down with your legs uncrossed, your arms at your sides or resting on your abdomen. Loosen any tight or constricting clothing. Close your eyes. Begin by inhaling slowly and deeply through your nostrils. Let the breath out through your nose slowly and completely. Continue breathing in this manner, allowing your abdomen to rise as you inhale and fall as you exhale. As you breathe allow yourself to relax.

Now imagine that you are in a high meadow. There are snow-capped mountains in the distance at each of the four corners. The meadow is surrounded by forest. It is a warm spring day. You are sitting in a circle of people that includes loved ones, friends, and healers. Everyone is there for a healing ceremony. Above the center of the circle you can feel a source of immense energy. The energy flows down toward each person on the edge of the circle, forming a cone. Feel the energy flow into your body. Reach out each of your hands and take the hands of the people to either side of you. Feel the energy coming from their hands. Close your eyes. Feel space and time expand.

If you have a problem or illness and wish to be healed, let go of the people's hands and move to the center of the circle. Let the circle move closer toward you, stopping when you feel comfortable. You are in a magic area now. You are lying in a shallow, bowl-shaped hollow in the middle of the circle. The area allows you to lie slightly below the people around you. Energy comes from the point above, down to the people in the circle where it is magnified greatly, and then it flows down the bowl into your body. If you wish, you can imagine that the people reach down into the bowl and touch you. Feel the energy come into your body from all the people. Receive the energy with love. Open yourself up to the gift of the energy. Let the energy fill your body and give you power. See the energy as light. Feel a tingling sensation as the energy flows into your body. Feel the energy concentrate near any area of illness. Let that area glow with healing energy. Picture the energy healing the illness. Picture viruses or unhealthy cells disappearing. Picture new, healthy tissue growing. See yourself as radiant and healed.

If you want to heal other people, picture them in the middle of the circle. See them clearly. Imagine that they are healthy, beautiful, and strong. Feel the energy coming from the point above down into your body. Feel the energy from the people to either side of you, whose hands you are holding. Feel the energy grow in your body. Now send the energy to the people you wish to heal. Give them the energy. Feel it flowing toward them. Picture their illness and watch as the energy heals it. See their illness disappearing. If you wish, you can imagine letting go of the people's hands and reaching down and touching the person you wish to be healed. As the energy passes through you let new energy fill you up. When you are finished, let any images of illness depart and picture yourself beautiful, healthy, and strong.

When you wish to return to your everyday state, gently move your feet and count slowly from one to three. You will return to your everyday state feeling relaxed and full of energy. Your body will feel as if it is in a comfortable, healing space. Each time you do this exercise you will relax more deeply and more easily. The feelings of relaxation will deepen, and the whole exercise will become more and more pleasurable.

. . .

By this time in a workshop, the group has usually bonded, and the people are supportive of each other. Many people feel the need for physical contact—hugging, therapeutic touch, and massage become more common experiences. A healing circle often forms spontaneously around people who are ill, in pain, emotionally upset, or simply in need of energy. At home, you can participate in these feelings by hugging family members or getting a massage from friends or healers. Most people who participate in healing circles find that their symptoms quickly show improvement. In one workshop a woman with cancer became anxious when she began to feel ill and experienced increased pain. She lay on the floor with the group around her in a circle. Each person in the group put a hand on her body and imagined that they were sending her healing energy. When the circle ended, the woman found she was more relaxed and her pain was gone. Each time I participate in a healing circle I'm amazed at the power of its results.

8

THE POWER: SPIRITUAL
TRANSFORMATION

In this, the last chapter of the book, we are nearing the end of our healing journey together. Here I will talk about power and life changes. We will use our inner strength to re-create our outer world. We will join inner and outer and will manifest the new creation. For me, the journey has been an exciting and creative one. Each day that I worked on this book was new and full of life and joy. The ideas were stimulating, the experiences enlightening and transformative. For me this year has been like a rebirth. I have allowed my natural interests and loves to draw me further into my work, and spontaneous visions have become more important in my healing techniques.

Every morning as I dreamed the book I became stronger, happier, and more whole. At the same time, the material was a challenge for me and took my full attention. Most of what I learn I try to use to create my life. I believe that my life is my work of art. Each thing I do is the art; I am the art. I strive to make my presence healing, each moment a healing gift to those around me. I work to make my house a piece of healing art, the place I see for my patients as a sacred space for healing.

Create your own life as a piece of healing art. Make each space you live in a sacred space of beauty and healing for you and everyone you meet and live with.

I live in the country far from crowded development. Animals surround my house. Patients see the animals as they come and the animals inform their healing process as spirit guides. This book was a high point in my life. Its channeled clear voice was a wonderful experience. The guided imagery exercises are beyond my personality, they are from a deep place of healing. Nancy gave me a huge gift by allowing the book to come through her with less than her normal input. She did her usual skilled and thoughtful writing. Her transparency was perfect for allowing the voice of this book to emerge. Her interests were not in shamanism and deep guided imagery; she lived in a world of love and faith in the intangible. I still love her deeply and honor her and the life and home we built together.

I hope that the exercises and material in the book will help you shape and transform your life and will help you heal yourself if you are ill. During the last several years my way of working with people who have illnesses has undergone change. I listen more, and while I listen, I go deep into my imagery space. I take my signals from each person and see an individual sacred geography that I share with that person. I feel in my body what I should do next. I increasingly use touch as a healing tool. I hope this book has given you a flavor of my work with people who are ill. My goal is to move increasingly toward visionary and sacred work that involves the soul as well as the mind and body.

Although the book's journey is coming to an end, the healing path is just beginning. Unlike a journey, a path never ends. It is made up of continuous moments. From this point in our path onward, we will continue to work and continue to let ourselves be transformed. We have started the work, and now we will let magic happen. The core of the work has been traveling inward, letting time and space dissolve, and living in energy and light. The question for each of us is "How can I do this when I am sick?" The answer is "Why not? How can I not?" Part of any illness is a loss of power and a subsequent loss of our own personal vision. When the body becomes ill, the disrupted energy of the body affects the mind and accentuates doubt and anxiety. When you go inside deeply, you contact the part that sees, regain your power and vision, and realize that you are still pure. When you go in deeper still, you connect to the All and realize that you are part of the One. In a metaphorical sense, you realize that you are like a god, that you live forever and are all-powerful. When you experience this book as one reader among many other readers, you will gain strength and are one. When you go inward, you contact the ancestors and get help.

If modern medicine invented a drug that made you feel powerful, in control, calm, and relaxed, it would be a major discovery. If its only side effects were feelings of well-being, that would be another advantage. It would be an even more remarkable medicine if it also relieved your discomfort and pain and often was capable of curing your illness and making you live longer. Going to your inner center provides such a medicine. To use this medicine, you don't have to understand or believe in the mind-body connection, in attitude and healing, in the effects of mental imagery, in God or a religion. You simply have to be interested enough to try this approach and experience the results.

There are forces that link us together and forces that separate us. The forces that link us together make us feel calm and powerful. The forces that separate us make us feel anxious and unsure. Health is generally increased by oneness, illness by separateness. Love is the main force that connects people and increases our power. Giving or receiving love immediately makes us feel wonderful. Its presence is transformative; it gives meaning to our lives. Love's parallel in nature is probably the force that holds molecules together. For a moment go inside and relive a moment of love. Notice how your body feels. Now pause a moment. Hate, on the other hand, is the force that separates. Whereas love builds, hate destroys. Briefly remember a moment of hate and remember how it made your body feel. Let it go; let love return. Beauty is a force that links. The experience of a rushing stream at dawn or a loved one's face draws us outside ourselves and connects us to the world around us. When we are ill, the outside world seems chaotic and confused. If we go inside, things become clearer, connections form, and we regain our power and vision. Strength can come from both inside and outside of us. When we regain our connections, we see that inside and outside are one. But to find this out we must go inside. Outside alone can be confusing; inside and outside together can heal.

This is a chapter about power. In our healing we regain our power and use it for transformation. In transformation we change and our worldview changes. Power enables us to alter our psychic orientation and see anew. This book encourages you to travel inside and regain your power. Everyone can do this; everyone can get better. By "getting better," I mean changing and improving ourselves, transforming each moment. Trust in yourself and the natural process that makes you better.

We can transform each moment, no matter what our state of health. When we do this, the body often follows and heals. By transforming our moments, we die; that is, our old self dies and a new self is born. Even in this age of scientific enlightenment, science cannot explain what death is. Science does not know whether there is a soul that lives on, or whether afterlife or reincarnation exists. Becoming ill puts us face-to-face with these questions and encourages us to explore and find our personal answers to them. Carlos Castaneda has written that death sits on our left shoulder at all times. This means that for all of us, no matter what our state of health, death is ever present. Although this is true, most people think of this only when they are ill. Researchers who have studied near-death experiences have found that subjects all report similar stories. Many people remember a vision of a tunnel with a light at the end. The feeling is one of peace and well-being. Many people also see loved ones and friends who are already dead beckoning to them. Whether this is true or merely a hallucination has not been proven by science.

For many people, a spiritual view of death is therapeutic. One cancer patient said, "You know the old saying 'There are no atheists in foxholes.' All of us are near or in the foxholes now." Working with or living with cancer patients, AIDS patients, and other people with life-threatening illnesses can be a gift to the helper. People who think about death can be more alive than those who are not ill. They deal constantly with what is real; they face the demons each day. To come out of that with a positive, clear vision, even occasionally, is true beauty and majesty. The realization that they give intensely the gift of life to all around them can be a source of strength for people who are severely ill.

Carl Jung believed that the concept of afterlife or reincarnation can make people feel better as they face death. Facing death is a momentous and profound experience, one that most people protect themselves from and avoid. However, facing death by itself is transforming. Simply looking at death allows us to be born again to new moments. It changes our moment-to-moment reality. In the study by David Spiegel that demonstrated life extension for breast cancer patients, the women in the support group spent a great deal of time talking about issues related to death. Dr. Spiegel has commented that he felt these discussions were of profound importance.

Why can't we fill each moment with magic and beauty? Our worldview prevents us from doing this because we are confused about what is real. When we can see that we are free, everything changes. When we can see that we are all one, we are released and see things anew. Is death real or figurative? If, as many believe, we have one life with many bodies, then death is always figurative. Science has never proven or understood what death is. Is our metaphorical rebirth with the new Self the same as death and rebirth into a new body? Seek these answers and believe what you feel. If an answer gives you strength and power, it is useful for your healing. If you have a life-threatening illness, you may find it useful to talk about death with a therapist who works in this field. Dealing with this material may free you to put all your energy into healing.

Seeing beyond the everyday world gives us back our power. Beyond to what? Beyond the everyday world, from separate to together, from apart to one, from concentrating on individual self to concentrating on universal Self, from selfish to Self-ish. We must die to our individual selves to be reborn to our Self. We must die to be reborn. The cycle must be finished. The renowned history-of-religions scholar Mircea Eliade has said that modern man thinks he is dying and sees nothingness all around him. This is an unnecessary tragedy. There is no use in fixating on nothingness unless it helps us see the absolute. Modern man can choose to see that he is dying and is one with everything that is around him. We must complete the rite of passage, not stop partway at death. We must continue to rebirth; we must return to the outer world and heal. We must finish the cycle with light and love. We can use our illness to be reborn in the moment. If illness is awful, it is also awe-ful; we can realize something positive from it. If before the illness our moments were full of worry or anger, but afterward our moments were radiant with love or peace, we have gotten *better.*

The key to changing our moments is changing our consciousness. In this book we do this by changing our basic attitudes, developing a personal myth, and journeying inward. We seek support from our inner center and our feeling of oneness with the universe. Through journeying inward, our view of the nature of reality can change; we can see we are one. Illness presents us with the choice of two philosophies. The first is "All is lost." The second is "All can be found." How does each of these make you feel? Which philosophy gives you power? We can choose the philosophy with which we view the world each minute. That is power, that is return of the soul. When we are healed, we *live* rather than live. One moment of *life* is better than an eternity of life.

I believe that all people can help themselves heal. At least in the moment, we can transform ourselves, and in the words of Joseph Campbell, we can find the still point of eternity around which everything revolves, and experience all as glorious. When this occurs, we are on the path toward wisdom. We realize that the Self is free, and its pain no longer belongs to us. We realize that "Thou art that." We are one, not separate from the universe, and the universe is for the benefit of the soul.

In the beginning of the book we did a welcoming ritual. This ritual started our journey inward and gave us the first feelings of the spaces to come. Now, as we come to the end of the book, I would like to do a closing ritual. This ritual will gather together our healing energies in symbolic form, so that we can continue on our healing path with increased energy. The ritual differs from the one in the beginning of the book in that it is a link between inner and outer, a purposeful attempt to bring the inner world outward. Because this ritual is an outer exercise, it is done differently.

Instead of closing your eyes, relaxing, and going inward, open your eyes, relax, and go outward. Take a walk around your house, your neighborhood, or a place in the country that you enjoy. Slow yourself down and feel the energy of the earth. Get healing from the earth; feel the sacred around you. The goal is to find an object that can contain or symbolize your healing powers. It may be a small statue, a piece of jewelry, a Zuni fetish, a picture, a rock, or a bouquet of flowers. You might want to create something of your own, such as a sculpture, a mask, or a decorated prayer stick. Whatever it is, it should be chosen because it speaks to you. It may be a new object or something you've had for years. Find a special place where you can make a little altar for this object. It may be outdoors or inside a building or even on your body. When you have found the object and its special place, put the object there as an offering. Let the energy of your visions flow into the object. Picture the object receiving healing energy from the universe, then directing the energy toward you. Make the object sacred. Mentally tell yourself and those you love what the object stands for in your life. Describe what healing energies it has and where the energy came from. Describe how you can use this object to increase your energy for healing. If you wish, you can prepare a short inner speech that will make an offering of this object to the world. The speech tells the world how the object helps you heal and reviews healing changes you plan to make in the outer world.

In a very real way, this is a book about dispelling ignorance and healing our Self. By "Self," we mean the whole of body, mind, and spirit. The paradox, of course, is that the Self is not sick; it simply needs to be discovered. And this discovery of the new Self that has been with us all along is like a rebirth. The new Self provides a better description of reality than the old. The emergence of this Self is like a rebirth because, to see it, our old self must die, that is, be transformed. Every moment that the old self is gone and the new Self is visible is a moment of dispelled ignorance. Dispelling ignorance involves the realization that we are or can be a new body and Self. The new Self is truly new. It is beyond attributes and understanding; it is timeless and spaceless. It is eternal and therefore beyond death. The extent to which we can grasp it is the extent of our power. As we allow it to emerge, we may not "know" it in the sense of logical thought, but we can feel it in the sense of oneness and power. I hope that through the hero's journey and myth, and with the help of inner figures, a glimpse of the new Self can be obtained. Once we have seen the new Self, we can bring it back in moments when we are ill.

Buddhists believe that the cause of suffering is attachment. When we become attached to people, ideas, or objects in the outer world, we experience suffering if our desires are not met. We become more and more involved with the objects of our desires until we identify with them, and this identification gives false reality to incidents in the outer world. The opposite of attachment is release. When we release our attachments and renounce the effects of our actions, we reenter the inner world and discover its timeless reality. This renunciation is basic to healing. Concentration on the process, and not desire for the fruits of the process, frees us from worry. To promote healing, we must release ourselves from worry about how the process is working and hold healing images not just for their effects but for the experience. When we use healing images, the healing process takes place by itself. Constantly checking to see if the process is working and constantly evaluating it are counterproductive; they create worry, which extinguishes the images. Doubt saps our power. Reenter the area where your power returns. It is very difficult to participate in the healing process without attachment to the final outcome. But each moment we can release ourself from the attachment, healing takes place more easily.

Attachment to our old self, to our conditionings, to the voices of parents and authority figures can produce guilt. The new self moves forward and in its timelessness doesn't worry about why something may have happened in the past. The path is experienced in here-and-now moments, and problems are dealt with directly. The old self, the old body, became ill because of the laws of cause and effect. The Hindus call these laws *karma*. Whether an illness is a result of genetics, environmental chemicals, microorganisms, poor dietary habits, or stress and attitude, some action that we participated in—purposefully or inadvertently—started the process of illness. The outer world and the old self interacted without any options, resulting in illness. We were who we were owing to our genetics, our upbringing, and the culture we were a part of; no blame was attached to their effects. When we become ill we participate in our illness, but we are blameless because we are simply who we are.

To heal, the new Self must create a new body. It must sweep clean and begin anew. For optimum effects, we need to participate in our healing, feel our power, and take control. We must use our strengths and move forward. We must release ourselves from blame but participate in the healing process. From this moment onward we can choose our attitudes and what we will concentrate on. Going beyond conditioning frees us from guilt. When we find that guilt causes worry, we can go inward, mentally list our strengths, increase our power, and review our support. In each workshop people talk about guilt. This is even more common now with AIDS patients, whose cultural burden is huge. People often blame themselves for being ill. They wonder if something they did made them ill. They speculate that chemicals, radiation, their own depression, or even a behavior pattern has caused their illness. If you feel this way, repeat to yourself the Taoist affirmation, "No blame." Guilt will not help you move forward. Forgive yourself. You don't have to hold yourself responsible for what you cannot control. You need not hold yourself personally responsible for your genetic background, your environment, your upbringing, or your lifelong, learned attitudes. Many professionals who work with cancer patients feel strongly that it is important that patients not blame themselves for causing their illness or not being able to cure it. At the same time, these professionals believe that patients are benefited if they participate in their healing. Thus, take control of your life now in whatever ways that you can. Remember, you are connected to the source. Your Self can make changes now that it is awake. You can participate in the present fully and help change the future. Accept the past, live the present, create the future.

Spiritual transformation creates our new Self and our new body. What makes us new? A new vision and a new attitude. I hope that this book has contributed to this process. A new vision allows us to see clearly across time and space, like an eagle in the mountains. The new sight, *in-sight,* increases our power and adds to our control. A personal myth gives our life meaning and changes our attitudes about the future. For moments we can feel new and, most important, feel light, radiance, and power.

What have we learned? I hope we have learned to look forward clearly and feel the energy of the world and our oneness with it. I hope this feeling betters each moment. When we are sick, we feel lost and weak. We need to let our inner Self fill us with light and power. We must go inside for the power, leaving behind the outer world with its attachments and its illusions. The inner world is more real, is closer to the truth, and will allow us to return to the outer world with strength. Healing flows from the new space in the inner world. It flows from the new Self to our new body. It re-creates a new body each moment that we can see our new Self.

To complete the circle, we must return to the outer world with strength. The final step in the hero's journey is the return. In the return, the hero brings his or her knowledge and understanding back from the sacred space to the everyday or profane world. In the inner world we find a boon, an elixir; we can even find a metaphor for everlasting life. We have glimpsed the truth of the oneness of the all and the eternal life of the soul. The hero's next task is to recross the threshold from inner to outer, the same threshold that we crossed when we entered into the sacred space.

This threshold is not crossed easily, but it must be traversed in order for the boon to be brought out. Bringing the power and knowledge from the inner world to the outer world is an essential part of healing. When this knowledge is brought out, it changes our consciousness, which in turn transforms our body. In the traditional hero's journey, bringing the gift back meant sharing the knowledge with others, which resulted in healing the earth, even the universe. The act of sharing this knowledge is an integral part of the hero's own healing.

Crossing the threshold is not easy. Inner knowledge is rationalized rapidly in the outer world and becomes meaningless. Often people do not comprehend inner knowledge and meet it with resentment. For a person who has been journeying inward, the outer world may look confusing and devoid of meaning. Some people even wonder if it is worth coming back. But life calls. From the inner world comes a feeling of peace, oneness, and power. The outer world can be seen as full of beauty, glory, movement, change, and action. Then with the loss of inner vision, the outer world once again becomes full of suffering, illness, and problems. Bringing the inner outward gives peace to mind and body. Healing occurs when images cross the threshold and become real in the outer world. The images allow action to occur; images heal the body. Images that are seen in the outer world as actions feed the soul and cause body, mind, and spirit to resonate. Each time images come outward, there is joy and fear: joy in the expression of our inner world, fear in having the images face the outer world.

Our task in going outward is to change our lives. In terms of healing, this is different for each person. Information from the inner world helps us to create our own personal healing path. With our guides, we can choose areas that intuitively seem important to our own healing. When we are ill, we are confronted with many choices concerning both conventional and complementary treatments. As people read and talk to physicians and friends, they will become aware of different treatments and lifestyle changes. Many healers working with cancer patients and people with life-threatening illnesses have found that people are more likely to get better when they have a role in choosing their therapies, have faith in them, and find them meaningful. By traveling inward, we can evaluate proposed therapies and find ones that feel right. Once people realize they have an interest in a particular treatment, the next step is to accomplish it in the outer world. When changes in medication, diet, exercise, stress, or support are made in conjunction with the doctor, a person's confidence and power grows. For example, a woman with cancer of the uterus was, at first, discouraged and depressed about her illness. But as she talked to people and started using imagery, she realized that there were many things that she could do to help herself get better in addition to having the surgery recommended by her doctor. She began by going on a vegetarian diet. Next she joined a women's support group to work on issues concerning her sexuality. During the time she was in the support group, her imagery changed and she started using ritual and dance to express her feelings about her illness. As time passed she paid much more attention to doing things that would give her pleasure: she bought a new car, she spent more time with her children, she traveled for the first time, and she made changes in her job.

Taking action in the outer world is the final step in the process. When the information derived from imagery is made real, a person's outer life changes. These life changes in the outer world feed back to the inner world and increase a person's feeling of power and strength. This increase in power makes it even easier for the person to act in the outer world, so the whole cycle reinforces itself and gains momentum.

In order for us to complete our journey, we must deal with the effects of reentering the outer world. It is said that even for a spiritual master who has glimpsed the essential nature of the cosmos, this is a difficult task. When we are nurtured and supported in the inner world, we often want to stay there. At the end of a workshop there is sadness in leaving the support of the sacred space and apprehension about facing problems in the "real" world. But when one knows that the soul is imperishable, one becomes imperishable. This knowledge is always difficult to carry across the threshold because it is wordless and often obliterated by the worries, attachments, and activity of the outer world. Throughout history spiritual masters have developed ways to keep inner knowledge alive in the outer world. One technique is the *cosmic dance*, which involves passing back and forth between inner and outer worlds rapidly in succession. This enables a person to glimpse knowledge and peace in the inner world and bring it forth to make changes in the outer world. As quickly as the inner knowledge is forgotten, the person must reimmerse him- or herself in the timeless inner world. Each time that we bring forth inner knowledge, we can do so more easily and quickly. The intense knowledge brought out changes our attitudes, and the attitudes change our actions. After a while there is a realization that the two worlds are actually one, that the inner world is a forgotten realm of the outer world and is always there.

The second major technique for keeping inner knowledge alive is *renunciation and release*. Attachments to objects and actions in the outer world make invisible the timeless knowledge of the inner world. Through renunciation, people are able to act in the outer world using the power of the inner world. The result of inner and outer being one is that people have the freedom to live, which makes them, in Joseph Campbell's words, the "champions of things becoming." This means that we permit the next moment to occur without becoming attached to or fighting it. Thus the world starts anew with every moment, the body is created anew, and we are healed.

The Discussion

In this, the last exercise of the book, we will use many of the techniques that we have learned in previous exercises. The goal of this exercise is to rest momentarily in the still point of eternity, around which everything revolves. This place is beyond attributes, beyond space and time, and even beyond images. The image is the vehicle for getting there, but the place itself is simply rest. It's like the moment between breathing in and breathing out. Since the space is beyond words, it is indescribable. But it is closer to silence than to noise. It is both light and dark, and it is without images. For most people it is probably impossible to experience this space for very long without serious preparation and spiritual guidance. In this exercise we hope that you can experience it for even a moment.

We will use many of the tools that we have learned in previous exercises to reach the space of silence. We will access the space through the inner world. In our imagination we will start with a leisurely walk. We will come to rest in our now familiar clearing. There we will come together as a group and join hands. We will then ascend, contact a guide, and walk into silence. If you wish, you can do this exercise in a group and actually touch physically while you do it. I've found that group energy and touch can make the exercise much more powerful. If you are ill, this exercise can give you rest and energy. The paradox of rest and energy creates healing. It's as if, in a space without words, opposites meet and illness is obliterated.

Finally we'll come back to the outer world. We'll cross the threshold and return to complete the circle. We will bring our inner knowledge outward; we will try to join the cosmic dance and move consciously back and forth across the world division that separates the timeless from the ephemeral. Do not rest in one spot, but lightly leap from one place to another without any fear.

The Exercises

Exercise 20—A Healing Mandala and Ascendant Vision.

Find a comfortable space where you will not be disturbed. Sit or lie down with your legs uncrossed, your arms at your sides or resting on your abdomen. Loosen any tight or constricting clothing. Close your eyes. Begin by inhaling slowly and deeply through your nostrils. Let the breath out through your nose slowly and completely. Continue breathing in this manner, allowing your abdomen to rise as you inhale and fall as you exhale. As you breathe allow yourself to relax.

Now imagine that you are walking on a soft dirt path at

dusk. The path is in the tropical hills, and it is warm and moist around you. The ground is cool and firm, and the path is clean of foliage. As you walk on the path you can feel the warm air touching your skin, you can smell the foliage and earth; occasionally you can feel plants to either side of the path touching your hands. The path climbs slowly. As it climbs, the air becomes cleaner and dryer, the foliage turns to grasses, and the ground becomes harder. The path now dips down into a gorge and goes across a wooden bridge. As you cross the bridge you can hear your feet make sounds on the wood like the tap on a drum. As you cross the bridge you get more and more relaxed. The closer you get to the other side of the bridge, the deeper your state of mind. The closer you get to the other side of the bridge, the stronger and more powerful you feel. The other side of the bridge is a different reality, where you see more clearly and are able to experience deeper realities. Across the bridge the path climbs gently through a thin forest; the light fades, and it becomes more difficult to see. You are going toward the last healing meeting during this group session. You feel excited and a little scared as you anticipate the experience.

Finally you enter a large clearing. You can see the sky above, with the first stars beginning to come out. The clearing is covered with grass. In the center there is a circle worn down by ages of use. The center of the circle is dark, and you can't see the ground there. At each of the four corners of the meadow, in the distance, is a high, snow-capped mountain. Above the meadow is a bright star. In the dark area in the center of the circle, the star is reflected mysteriously. You walk up to the circle and sit down. People come from the path you're on and sit around the circle with you. In the fading light you can barely recognize relatives, dear friends, and healers that have been on the journey with you. An elder speaks. The elder asks you to join hands and feel the circle become a ring of energy. Feel the energy from the star flow down in a cone into the circle of people. Let this energy fill your body, flow to the reflection in the center of the circle, and move back to the star. The elder thanks you for participating in the healing and hopes that you will experience the place of silence.

The elder tells you to stand up and walk toward the center of the circle. The elder instructs the group to lie on their backs with their heads facing toward the center of the circle and their feet pointing outward from the center. Anyone who feels ill should place themselves toward the center. Everyone should touch the other people on the sides of their bodies. The group forms a flat pinwheel-like mandala. The reflection in the center of the circle can be seen below the heads that are toward the center. The elder tells you to close your eyes.

Now you become aware of a spiral of light that goes from the outside of the circle toward the center. The spiral is reddish orange and seems to be alive. The spiral lies on the disc of people but is not part of them. Now the spiral starts to rotate. It starts to turn slowly in a clockwise direction. As it turns, the entire group of people can be seen to rotate with it. The spiral spins slowly. As the spiral spins it seems to rise slowly off the ground. As it rises you can feel yourself rise with it. The disc of people and the spiral slowly spin and rise. You rise out of the clearing, above the forest, above the mountains, above the earth.

The disc continues to spin and rise. As it rises you become more and more relaxed. Your body becomes lighter. You can feel energy moving within your body. The disc rises and spins, higher and higher. Finally the spinning begins to slow. The disc spins more and more slowly. The disc stops spinning. The elder asks you to stand. Everyone stands.

You are on a flat plane in space. The plane supports you but cannot be seen. The space around you glows with a soft light. You can feel the light pass through your body and give you energy. Everyone starts walking toward a light area in the distance. As you walk you feel someone next to you take your hand. You are now accompanied by a guide. The guide does not speak. You feel wonderful energy flowing from the guide into your body. The guide makes you feel stronger but at the same time protects and leads you.

The area of light ahead gets closer. You can now see that it is a large gate. The gate glows with bright white light. On either side of the gate is an animallike figure. Each person and his or her guide pass through the gate. You pass along the stairway that glows and leads through the doorway. As you come up to the doorway you can see nothing beyond it. As the figures in front of you go through, they disappear. The guide touches you, and you feel strong and powerful.

You go through the doorway, and all disappears. Your body comes apart and breaks into the tiniest pieces, and the pieces fly off in all directions. All feelings of touch, smell, hearing, and sight fly off in all directions. There is simply silence and the perception of energy. The perception is not you but is everything. Energy is everywhere. You are everywhere. You are one with the energy of the universe. Rest in this place as long as you wish. Feel the oneness with the forces of the universe. Feel the exhilarating sense of peace.

Now feel your body come back together. See and feel the parts and pieces rapidly coming from everywhere and reassembling as a new, energized body. As each piece comes toward you its energy increases. It's purified and made holy. Let your body come together and absorb the energy of the universe. Feel your new body in its power and radiance.

Now look around you. You again are on a plane. The light of the plane passes through you and gives you energy. Again your guide's hand touches yours, and you start walking back toward the place where you arrived. You feel the wonderful energy flowing from the guide's hand into your body. You are now at peace, powerful, confident, and strong. You see others walking with you toward the arrival point. Their radiance and beauty fill you with love.

You leave your guide and lie down with others in a circle with your head facing the center and your arms touching the people next to you. You become aware of a spiral of light that goes from the outside of the circle toward the center. The spiral lies on the disc of people but is not part of them. Now the spiral starts to rotate. It starts to turn slowly in a counterclockwise direction. The spiral spins slowly. As the spiral turns, it drops down. As it drops, you can feel yourself drop with it. The disc and spiral drop down toward earth, toward the mountains, toward the forests, toward the clearing. Finally the spinning begins to slow. The disc spins more and more slowly and finally stops spinning.

You are on the ground in the clearing. You stand and feel the energy of the others around you. You touch the others and say good-bye. Feel the love flowing from your body into the others and from their bodies into you. You see your path out of the clearing and start toward it. The path leads down toward a bridge, crosses it, and then climbs slowly. The path continues through the grassy area and ends in the room where you started.

When you wish to return to your everyday state, gently move your feet and count slowly from one to three. You will return to your everyday state feeling relaxed, comfortable, and full of energy. Your body will feel as if it is in a comfortable, healing space. Each time you do this exercise you will relax more deeply and more easily. The feelings of relaxation will deepen, and the whole exercise will become more and more pleasurable.

Open your eyes and see the room. See the beautiful things that surround you in your life. Feel power, strength, and confidence. Close your eyes again: feel the peace and power from inside you. Open your eyes: see the glory and beauty that surround you. Bring your vision outward. Think of changes you can make in your outer world. Close your eyes again: feel the power, peace, and confidence in you. Open your eyes: bring your inner vision outward.

As you leave this book, I hope that you take some of it with you in your everyday view of the world. I hope that it helps you to access your inner world for healing and helps you to bring your knowledge outward. I hope that it gives you power in moments of weakness and courage in moments of fear. I hope that it relieves suffering and makes you live longer. I say good-bye to you in thanks. Thank you for your presence and power. I feel your energy as a reader, and it is a gift. Thank you. Go in peace and health.

NOTES

CHAPTER 1. THE AWAKENING

1. Tapes can be found in the New Age section of bookstores and record stores. My favorites include tapes by Don Campbell, Kay Gardner, and Mike Rowland.

CHAPTER 2. THE VEHICLE: REVERIE STATES

1. For excellent bibliographies on the effects of mind states on illness, see books in the bibliography by Justice, Ornstein and Sobel, and Pelletier and Herzing.
2. Schrödinger, E. 1969. *What Is Life?* Cambridge University Press, p. 145.

CHAPTER 3. THE JOURNEY: ATTITUDES AND PERSONAL MYTHS

1. Jung, C. G. 1964. *Man and His Symbols,* Doubleday & Co., p. 161.
2. Ornstein, R., and Sobel, D. 1987. *The Healing Brain,* Simon & Schuster, p. 206.
3. Kaplan, M. 1986. "Social Support and Health," *Medical Care* 15:47.
4. Jung, C. G. 1963. *Memories, Dreams, Reflections,* Vintage Books, p. 252.
5. Campbell, J. 1973. *Myths to Live By,* Bantam Books, p. 89.
6. Ibid., p. 136.
7. Ibid., p. 136.
8. Ibid., p. 136.

CHAPTER 4. INNER GUIDES: HELPING FIGURES

1. Eliade, M. 1964. *Shamanism,* Princeton University Press, p. 107.
2. Jung, C. G. 1963. *Memories, Dreams, Reflections,* Vintage Books, p. 179.
3. Ibid., p. 181.
4. Ibid., p. 183.
5. Ibid., p. 189.

CHAPTER 5. THE LIGHT

1. Bolle, K. 1979. *The Bhagavadgita,* University of California Press, p. 129.

BIBLIOGRAPHY

Achterberg, J. 1985. *Imagery and Healing.* Shambhala.

Ader, R. 1981. *Psychoneuroimmunology.* Academic Press.

Antonovsky, A. 1984. "A Sense of Coherence as a Determinant of Health," *Behavioral Health.* J. Matarazzo, ed., John Wiley & Sons.

Baider, L., Uziely, B., and De-Nour, K. 1994. "Progressive Muscle Relaxation and Guided Imagery in Cancer Patients." *General Hospital Psychiatry,* 16: 340–347.

Bandura, A. 1985. "Catecholamine Secretion as a Function of Perceived Coping Self-Efficacy." *Journal of Consulting and Clinical Psychology* 53:3:406.

Benjamin, H. 1987. *From Victim to Victor.* Dell Books.

Blofeld, J. 1970. *The Tantric Mysticism of Tibet.* Prajna Press.

Bolle, K. 1979. *The Bhagavadgita.* University of California Press.

Borysenko, J. 1987. *Minding the Body, Mending the Mind.* Addison-Wesley.

Brown-Saltzman, K. 1997. "Replenishing the Spirit by Meditative Prayer and Guided Imagery." *Seminars in Oncology Nursing* 13(4):255–9.

Campbell, J. 1967. *The Hero with a Thousand Faces.* Meridian Books.

———. 1973. *Myths to Live By.* Bantam.

———. 1976. *The Masks of God: Oriental Mythology.* Penguin.

———. 1976. *The Masks of God: Primitive Mythology.* Penguin.

———. 1986. *The Inner Reaches of Outer Space.* Alfred Van Der Marck.

Carroll, D., and Seers, K. 1998. "Relaxation for the Relief of Chronic Pain: A Systematic Review." *Journal of Advanced Nursing,* 27: 476–87.

Castaneda, C. 1981. *The Eagle's Gift.* Pocket Books.

Clouse, M. 1999. "Alternative Medicine in Radiology." *Academic Radiology,* 6: 455–6.

Dossey, L. 1988. "The Rediscovery of the Mind." *Advances* 5:3:73.

———. 2000. "Hypnosis: A Window into the Soul of Healing." *Alternative Therapies in Health and Medicine,* 6(2):12–17, 102–110.

Eliade, M. 1957. *Myths, Dreams, and Mysteries.* Harper & Row.

———. 1957. *The Sacred and the Profane.* Harcourt Brace & World.

———. 1958. *Rites and Symbols of Initiation.* Harper & Row.

———. 1958. *Yoga Immortality and Freedom.* Pantheon.

———. 1969. *The Two and the One.* Harper & Row.

———. 1972. *Shamanism.* Princeton University Press.

Eller, L. S. 1999. "Guided Imagery Interventions for Symptom Management." *Annual Review of Nursing Research.* (vol. 1). New York: Springer Publishing Company.

Evans-Wentz, W. Y. 1958. *Tibetan Yoga and Secret Doctrines.* Oxford University Press.

Fawzy, F. I., Kemeny, M. E., Fawzy, N. W., Elashoff, R., Morton, D., Cousins, N., and Fahey, J. L. 1990. "A Structured Psychiatric Intervention for Cancer Patients: II. Changes over Time in Immunological Measures." *Archives of General Psychiatry,* 47: 729–35.

Feldman, C. S., and Salzberg, H. C. 1990. "The Role of Imagery in the Hypnotic Treatment of Adverse Reactions to Cancer Therapy." *Journal of South Carolina Medical Association* 86(5):303–6.

Fernandez, E., and Turk, D. C. 1989. "The Utility of Cognitive Coping Strategies for Altering Pain Perception: A Meta-Analysis." *Pain,* 28: 123–35.

Fick, L. J., Lang, E. V., Logan, H. L., Lutgendorf, S., and Benotsch, E. G. 1999. "Imagery Content During Nonpharmacologic Analgesic in the Procedure Suite: Where Your Patients Would Rather Be." *Academic Radiology,* 6, 457–63.

Fox, M. 1988. *The Coming of the Cosmic Christ.* Harper & Row.

Hall, H. R. 1983. "Hypnosis and the Immune System." *Journal of Clinical Hypnosis* 25:2:92.

Harner, M. 1982. *The Way of the Shaman.* Bantam.

Harris, W. S., et al. 1999. "A Randomized, Controlled Trial of the Effects of Remote, Intercessory Prayer on Outcomes in Patients Admitted to the Coronary Care Unit." *Archives of Internal Medicine* 159(19):2273,

Horrigan, B. 2002. Marty Rossman, M.D., "Imagery: The Body's Natural Language for Healing." *Alternative Therapies in Health and Medicine,* 8, (1): 81–9.

Jacobson, E. 1965. *How to Relax and Have Your Baby.* McGraw-Hill.

Jahn, G. 1987. *Margins of Reality.* Harcourt, Brace Jovanovich.

Jung, C. 1961. *Memories, Dreams, Reflections.* Vintage Books.

———. 1964. *Man and His Symbols.* Doubleday & Co.

Justice, B. 1987. *Who Gets Sick.* Tarcher.

Kabat-Zinn, J., et al. 1998. "Influence of a Mindfulness Meditation-based Stress Reduction Intervention on Rates of Skin Clearing in Patients with Moderate to Severe Psoriasis Undergoing Phototherapy (UVB) and Photochemotherapy (PUVA)." *Psychosomatic Medicine* 60(5):625–32.

Klaus, M., and Kennell, J. 1982. *Parent-Infant Bonding.* C. V. Mosby.

Kobasa, S. 1981. "Personality and Constitution as Mediators in the Stress-Illness Relationship." *Journal of Health and Social Behavior* 22:368.

Kolcaba, K., and Fox, C. 1999. "The Effects of Guided Imagery on Comfort of Women with Early Stage Breast Cancer Undergoing Radiation Therapy." *Oncology Nursing Forum,* 26(1):67–72.

Krup, M. 1988. *Current Medical Diagnosis and Treatment*. Appleton and Lang.

Kwekkeboom, K., Huseby-Moore, K., and Ward, S. 1998. "Imagining Ability and the Effective Use of Guided Imagery." *Research in Nursing and Health*, 21 (30), 189–98.

Lang, E.V., et al. (2000). "Adjunctive Non-pharmacological Analgesia for Invasive Medical Procedures: A Randomized Trial." *Lancet*, 355: 1486–90.

Lee, R., and DeVore, I. 1976. *Kalahari Hunter-Gatherers*. Harvard University Press.

LeShan, L. 1989. *Cancer as a Turning Point*. E. P. Dutton.

Levine, S. 1974. *Meetings at the Edge*. Doubleday and Co.

Locke, S. 1986. *The Healer Within*. New American Library.

Loder, J. E. 1989. *The Transforming Moment*. Colorado Springs: Helmers & Howard.

Lovelock, J. E. 1979. *Gaia*. Oxford University Press.

Luthe, W. 1970. *Autogenic Therapy*. Grune & Stratton.

Matthews-Simonton, S., and Simonton, C. 1978. *Getting Well Again*. Bantam.

McClelland, D. 1985. "Healing Motives: An Interview with David McClelland." *Advances* 2:29.

Milton, D. 1998. "Alternative and Complementary Therapies: Integration into Cancer Care." *American Association of Holistic Nursing*, 46(9):454–61.

Moyers, B. 1993. *Healing and the Mind*. New York: Doubleday.

Muktananda, S. 1980. *Meditate*. State University of New York Press.

Myss, C. 1996. *Anatomy of the Spirit*. New York: Three Rivers Press.

Naprastek, B. 1994. *Staying Well with Guided Imagery*. New York: Warner Books, Inc.

Nilsson, L. 1974. *Behold Man*. Little, Brown.

Nuckolls, K. 1972. "Psychosocial Assets, Life Crisis and the Prognosis of Pregnancy." *American Journal of Epidemiology* 95:431.

O'Leary, A. 1985. "Self-Efficacy and Health." *Behavior, Research and Therapy* 23:437.

Ornstein, R., and Sobel, D. 1987. *The Healing Brain*. Simon & Schuster.

Oyle, I. 1974. *The Healing Mind*. Celestial Arts.

Pelletier, K., and Herzing, D. 1988. "Psychoneuroimmunology: Toward a Mindbody Model." *Advances* 5:1:27.

Pert, C. 1986. "The Wisdom of the Receptors: Neuropeptides, the Emotions, and Bodymind." *Advances* 3:3:8.

Richardson, M. A., et al. 1997. "Coping, Life Attitudes, and Immune Responses to Imagery and Group Support after Breast Cancer Treatment." *Alternative Therapies in Health and Medicine*, 3(5):62–70.

Rossman, M. 1987. *Healing Yourself*. Walker and Co.

Samuels, M., and Bennett, H. 1972. *The Well Body Book*. Random House–Bookworks.

———. 1973. *Spirit Guides*. Random House–Bookworks.

———. 1974. *Be Well*. Random House–Bookworks.

———. 1982. *Well Body, Well Earth*. Sierra Club.

Samuels, M., and Lane, M. R. 2000. *Spirit Body Healing: Using Your Mind's Eye to Unlock the Medicine Within*. New York: John Wiley & Sons.

Samuels, M., and Samuels, N. 1975. *Seeing with the Mind's Eye*. Random House–Bookworks.

———. 1988. *The Well Adult*. Summit Books.

Schneider, J., et al. 1983. "The Relationship of Mental Imagery to White Blood Cell (Neutrophil) Function." Uncirculated monograph, Michigan State University College of Medicine.

Shlain, L. 1998. *The Alphabet Versus the Goddess*. New York: Penquin/ Arkana.

Siegel, B. S. 1986. *Love, Medicine & Miracles*. Harper & Row.

———. 1989. *Peace, Love and Healing: Bodymind Communication and the Path to Self-healing: An Exploration*. New York: Harper Perennial.

Simonton, S. S., and Sherman, A. C. (1998). "Psychological Aspects of Mindbody Medicine: Promises and Pitfalls from Research with Cancer Patients." *Alternative Therapies*, 4 (4): 50–64.

Siuta, J. 1996. "The Imagination Inventory and Its Correlates with Imagery and Hypnotizability." *American Journal of Clinical Hypnosis*, 39(2):115–25.

Sloman, R. 1995. "Relaxation and the Relief of Cancer Pain." *Nursing Clinics of North America*, 30 (4): 697–709.

Smith, H. 2001. *Why Religion Matters: The Fate of the Human Spirit in an Age of Disbelief*. San Francisco: HarperSanFrancisco.

Smith, M.C., Holcombe, J. K., and Stullenbarger, E. 1994. "A Meta-analysis of Intervention Effectiveness for Symptom Management in Oncology Nursing Research." *Oncology Nursing Forum*, 21(7):1201–9.

Spiegel, D., and Bloom, J. R. 1983. "Group Therapy and Hypnosis Reduce Metastatic Breast Carcinoma Pain." *Psychosomatic Medicine*, 45(4):333–9.

Spiegel, D., Bloom, J. R., Kraemer, H. C., & Gottheil, E. 1989. "Effect of Psychosocial Treatment on Survival of Patients with Metastatic Breast Cancer." *The Lancet*, 2: 888–91.

Spiegel, D., et al. 1989. "Effect of Psychosocial Treatment on Survival of Women with Metastatic Breast Cancer." *Lancet* 2(8668):888–91.

Sprenkle, D. H., and Moon, S. M. 1996. "Toward Pluralism in Family Therapy Research." In D. H. Sprenkle and S. M. Moon (Eds.), *Research Methods in Family Therapy*. New York: Guilford Press.

Sugarman, J., and Burk, L. 1998. "Physicians' Ethical Obligations Regarding Alternative Medicine." *The Journal of the American Medical Association*, 280: 1623–5.

Swimme, B. 1984. *The Universe Is a Green Dragon*. Bear & Co.

Syrjala, K. L., Donaldson, G. W., Davis, M. W., Kippes, M. E., Carr, J. E. 1995. "Relaxation and Imagery and Cognitive-behavioral Training

Reduce Pain during Cancer Treatment: A Controlled Clinical Trial." *Pain* 63(2):189–98.

Tart, C. 1972. *Altered States of Consciousness.* Doubleday and Co.

Thomas, C., et al. 1979. "Family Attitudes in Youth as Potential Predictors of Cancer." *Psychosomatic Medicine* 41:287.

Tope, D. M., Ahles, T. A., and Silberfarb, P. M. 1998. "Psycho-oncology: Psychological Well-being as One Component of Quality of Life." In G. A. Fava and H. Freyberger (Eds.), *Handbook of Psychosomatic Medicine* (pp. 341–372). Connecticut: International Universities Press.

Tusek, D., Church, J. M., Fazio, V. W. 1997. "Guided Imagery as a Coping Strategy for Perioperative Patients." *AORN Journal* 66(4):644–9.

Tusek, D. L., Church, J. M., Strong, S. A. , Grass, J. A., Fazio, V. W. 1997. "Guided Imagery: A Significant Advance in the Care of Patients Undergoing Elective Colorectal Surgery." *Diseases of the Colon and Rectum* 40(2):172–8.

Tusek, D. L., Cwynar, R., Cosgrove, D. M. 1997. "Effect of Guided Imagery on Length of Stay, Pain and Anxiety in Cardiac Surgery Patients." *Journal of Cardiovascular Management* 10(2):22–8.

Walker, L. G., et al. 1999. "Psychological, Clinical and Pathological Effects of Relaxation Training and Guided Imagery during Primary Chemotherapy." *British Journal of Cancer* 80(1–2):262–8.

Wallace, K. G. 1997. "Analysis of Recent Literature Concerning Relaxation and Imagery Interventions For Cancer Pain." *Cancer Nursing* 20(2):79–87. Review.

Weil, A. 1997. *Sound Mind, Sound Body: Music for Healing with Andrew Weil, M.D.* (CD). New York: Upaya.

Wilhelm, R. 1969. *The Secret of the Golden Flower.* Routledge & Kegan Paul.

Wolman, R. N. 2001. *Thinking with Your Soul: Spiritual Intelligence and Why It Matters.* New York: Harmony Books.

Woodman, M. 1982. *Addiction to Perfection.* Inner City Books.

Wyngaarden, J. 1989. *Cecil Textbook of Medicine.* W. B. Saunders.

Zachariae, R., Kristensen, J. S., Ellegaard, J., Metze, E. and Hokland, P. 1990. "Effect of Psychological Intervention in the Form of Relaxation and Guided Imagery on Cellular Immune Function of Normal Healthy Subjects." *Psychotherapy and Psychosomatics,* 54: 32–9.

INDEX

Printed in the USA
CPSIA information can be obtained
at www.ICGtesting.com
JSHW012023140824
68134JS00033B/2844

9 780471 459088